# ONCOLOGY

**International Journal of Cancer Research and Treatment**

Founded 1948 as 'Oncologia' by H.R. Schinz
Continued by V. Richards (1967–1975), H. Wrba (1976–1992)



KARGER

Printed in Switzerland
on acid-free paper by
Druckerei Schüler AG, Biel

Appears bimonthly:
1 volume per year (6 issues)

# ONCOLOGY

**Submission:** Only original papers written in English are considered and should be sent to:

S. Karger AG
Editorial Dept. 'Oncology'
P.O. Box
CH-4009 Basel (Switzerland)

Manuscripts should be submitted in triplicate (with three sets of illustrations of which one is an original), typewritten double-spaced on one side of the paper, with a wide margin.

**Conditions:** All manuscripts are subject to editorial review. The editors reserve the right to improve style and, if necessary, return the manuscript for re-writing to the author. Submission of an article for publication implies the transfer of the copyright from the author to the publisher upon acceptance. Accepted papers become the permanent property of 'Oncology' and may not be reproduced by any means, in whole or in part, without the written consent of the publisher. It is the author's responsibility to obtain permission to reproduce illustrations, tables, etc. from other publications.

**Arrangement**

*Title page:* The first page of each paper should indicate the title (main title underlined), the authors' names, and the institute where the work was conducted. A short title for use as running head as well as the full address of the author to whom correspondence should be sent are also required.

*Full address:* The exact postal address complete with postal code must be given at the bottom of the title page. Please also supply Phone and Fax numbers.

*Key words:* For indexing purposes, a list of 3-10 key words in English is essential.

*Abstract:* Each paper needs an abstract of up to 10 lines.

*Small type:* Paragraphs which can or must be set in smaller type (case histories, test methods, etc.) should be indicated with a 'p' (petit) in the margin on the left-hand side.

*Footnotes:* Avoid footnotes. When essential, they are numbered consecutively and typed at the foot of the appropriate page.

*Tables and illustrations:* Tables and illustrations (both numbered in Arabic numerals) should be prepared on separate sheets. Tables require a heading and figures a legend, also prepared on a separate sheet. For the reproduction of illustrations, only good drawings and original photographs can be accepted; negatives or photocopies cannot be used. When possible, group several illustrations on one block for reproduction (max. size 181 × 223 mm) or provide crop marks. On the back of each illustration, indicate its number, the author's name, and 'top'. Color illustrations are reproduced at the author's expense.

*References:* In the text identify references by Arabic numerals [in square brackets]. Material submitted for publication but not yet accepted should be noted as 'unpublished data' and not be included in the reference list. The list of references should include only those publications which are cited in the text. Do not alphabetize; number references in the order in which they are first mentioned in the text. The surnames of the authors followed by initials should be given. There should be no punctuation other than a comma to separate the authors. Cite all authors, 'et al' is not sufficient. Abbreviate journal names according to the Index Medicus system. (Also see International Committee of Medical Journal Editors: Uniform requirements for manuscripts submitted to biomedical journals. Br Med J 1988;296:401-405.)

*Examples*

*(a) Papers published in periodicals:* Kauffman HF, van der Heide S, Beaumont F, Blok H, de Vries K: Class-specific antibody determination against *Aspergillus fumigatus* by means of the enzyme-linked immunosorbent assay. III. Comparative study: IgG, IgA, IgM ELISA titers, precipitating antibodies and IgE binding after fractionation of the antigen. Int Arch Allergy Appl Immunol 1986;80:300-306.

*(b) Monographs:* Matthews DE, Farewell VT: Using and Understanding Medical Statistics. Basel, Karger, 1985.

*(c) Edited books:* Hardy WD Jr, Essex M: FeLV-induced feline acquired immune deficiency syndrome: A model for human AIDS; in Klein E (ed): Acquired Immunodeficiency Syndrome. Prog Allergy. Basel, Karger, 1986, vol 37, pp 353-376.

*Further details:* Authors may consult our leaflet 'Rules for the Preparation of Manuscripts', available on request from the Publisher, S. Karger AG, P.O. Box, CH-4009 Basel (Switzerland).

**Page charges:** There is no page charge for papers of 3 or fewer printed pages (including tables, illustrations and references). Each additional complete or partial page is charged to the author at SFr. 225.– / US$ 150.00. The allotted size of a paper is equal to approx. 9 manuscript pages (including tables, illustrations and references).

**Galley proofs:** Unless indicated otherwise, galley proofs are sent to the first-named author and should be returned with the least possible delay. Alterations made in galley proofs, other than the correction of printer's errors, are charged to the author. No page proofs are supplied.

**Reprints:** Order forms and a price list are sent with the galley proofs. Orders submitted after the issue is printed are subject to considerably higher prices. Allow five weeks from date of publication for delivery of reprints.

KARGER

General Information

ONCOLOGY

**Publication data:** 'Oncology' is published 6 times annually. Volume 51 with 6 issues appears in 1994.

**Subscription rates:** Subscriptions run for a full calendar year. Prices are given per volume.

*Personal subscription:*

*Subscription + postage and handling*
SFr. 558.60 + SFr. 16.80 Europe
SFr. 558.60 + SFr. 25.20 Overseas
US$ 373.10 + US$ 16.80
(Must be in the name of, billed to, and paid by an individual. Order must be marked 'personal subscription'.)

*Institutional subscription:*

*Subscription + postage and handling*
SFr. 798.– + SFr. 24.– Europe
SFr. 798.– + SFr. 36.– Overseas
US$ 533.00 + US$ 24.00

*Airmail postage:* SFr. 36.–, US$ 30.00. (Extra per volume.)

*Microform edition:* SFr. 399.00, US$ 266.50. (Available exclusively to subscribers of the paper edition.)

**Advertising:** Correspondence and rate requests should be addressed to the Publisher.

**Subscription orders:** Orders can be placed at agencies, bookstores, directly with the Publisher S. Karger AG, P.O. Box, CH–4009 Basel (Switzerland) or with any of the following distributors:

*Deutschland:* S. Karger GmbH, Postfach D–79095 Freiburg

*France:* Librairie Luginbühl
36, bd de Latour-Maubourg, F–75007 Paris

*Great Britain, Ireland:* S. Karger Publishers
11 Ravenscroft Road
Beckenham, Kent BR3 4TP

*USA:* S. Karger Publishers, Inc.
26 West Avon Road, P.O. Box 529
Farmington, CT 06085

*India, Bangladesh, Sri Lanka:*
S. Karger India Subscription Agency
B–5/132 Safdarjung Enclave
New Delhi-110029

*Japan:* Katakura Libri, Inc.
36-9 Hongo 3-chome, Bunkyo-ku, Tokyo 113

**Change of address:** Both old and new address should be sent to the subscription source.

**Single issues and back volumes:** Information can be obtained through the Publisher.

**Bibliographic indices:** This journal is regularly listed in bibliographic services, including *Current Contents®*.

**Book Reviews:** Books are accepted for review by special agreement.



KARGER

# Role of Cytokines in Cancer Treatment

Guest Editor
*F. Takaku,* Tokyo

15 figures and 21 tables, 1994

KARGER

S. Karger
Medical and Scientific Publishers
Basel · Freiburg · Paris · London
New York · New Delhi · Bangkok
Singapore · Tokyo · Sydney

Drug Dosage
The authors and the publisher have exerted every effort to ensure that drug selection and dosage set forth in this text are in accord with current recommendations and practice at the time of publication. However, in view of ongoing research, changes in government regulations, and the constant flow of information relating to drug therapy and drug reactions, the reader is urged to check the package insert for each drug for any change in indications and dosage and for added warnings and precautions. This is particularly important when the recommended agent is a new and/or infrequently employed drug.


Printed in Switzerland on acid-free paper by
Graphische Anstalt Schüler AG, Biel
ISBN 3-8055-5948-8

# Contents

# Introductory Remarks

*F. Takaku*

Tokyo

Cytokines are proteins regulating a wide spectrum of physiological processes including the growth and differentiation of cells of the immune and hematopoietic systems. Some cytokines such as interferons have direct cytotoxic activity on cancer cells. Recent developments in biotechnology have made it possible to produce sufficient quantities of cytokines of suitable purity for clinical use, including cancer treatment.

Interferons were the first cytokines used in cancer treatment, and they are now the first-line drug for the treatment of chronic myelogenous leukemia and hairy cell leukemia. Meanwhile combining interferons with cytotoxic drugs is a challenging clinical research project in cancer treatment. Although interleukin-2 has limited clinical applications in cancer therapy, this cytokine has many interesting activities which necessitate further research.

Hematopoietic growth factors, which are mainly used as adjuvants in cancer treatment to reconstitute the bone marrow after chemotherapy, are expected to accelerate the release of hematopoietic stem cells into peripheral blood and may then be used for peripheral blood stem cell transplantation.

This special issue of *Oncology* has been planned to introduce the latest trends in the clinical application of these cytokines in cancer treatment. It is the editor's hope that through the articles that follow, readers will become acquainted with the most recent knowledge acquired in this field.

Oncology 1994;51:123–128

*Fumimaro Takaku*

National Medical Center, Tokyo, Japan

# Clinical Application of Cytokines for Cancer Treatment

**Key Words**
Cancer treatment
Interferon
Interleukin-2
Hematopoietic growth factors

**Abstract**
As the introduction to a special issue of *Oncology* on the role of cytokines for cancer treatment, this article summarizes their various current uses. Interferons, interleukin-2 and hematopoietic factors are extensively used for the treatment of hematopoietic as well as nonhematopoietic malignancies, either as the main therapeutic agents or as an adjuvant. Combined usage of several cytokines, or cytokines and chemotherapeutic agents has been tried. Research on gene therapy using cytokines is in progress and expected to become a future modality of cytokine usage in cancer treatment.

Cytokines are proteins produced by various cells to regulate a wide spectrum of physiological processes including the regulation of growth and differentiation of the cells of the immune and hematopoietic system. Cytokines are also involved in the pathophysiology of various human diseases. These proteins thus have therapeutic potential in human diseases including cancer, and recent biotechnology developments have made it possible to produce recombinant cytokines of satisfactory purity in sufficient quantity to be used for clinical purposes.

## Interferons

Among the cytokines, interferons (IFNs) were the first used for cancer treatment. IFN-α which has at least 16 subtypes has been most widely used in the last several years to treat patients with hairy-cell leukemia, chronic myelogenous leukemia, multiple myeloma, certain non-Hodgkin's lymphomas, AIDS-associated Kaposi's sarcoma, renal cell carcinoma, malignant melanoma, and viral hepatitis. It has also been used for the intralesional treatment of venereal warts.

Hairy cell leukemia was the first hematological malignancy for which the specific efficacy of IFN-α was identified [1]. Overall, approximately 90% of patients will benefit symptomatically from IFN-α therapy. IFN, however, does not cure hairy cell leukemia, and up to 50% of patients will relapse after treatment discontinuation. Most relapsed patients will respond to retreatment with IFN-α, and a recent paper reported that the continuous administration of IFN-α induced a long survival up to 6 years [2] in 82% of patients with this leukemia.

The effectiveness of IFN-α for chronic myelogenous leukemia was recognized in the early 1980s. It was first recognized that treatment with partially purified native IFN-α could induce a hematological remission in patients with chronic myelogenous leukemia [3]. Further clinical study on chronic myelogenous leukemia revealed an unexpected diminution or even elimination of Philadelphia-positive cells from the patient's bone marrow [4]. This cytogenetic activity of IFN-α in chronic myelogenous leukemia was later confirmed by other groups using native as well as recombinant products. Although similar cytogenetic responses can occur after aggressive chemotherapy, they are generally quite brief. Administration of IFN-α,

Fumimaro Takaku, MD
International Medical Center of Japan
1-21-1 Toyama-cho
Shinjuku-ku
Tokyo 162 (Japan)


0030–2414/94/0512–0123
$5.00/0

therefore, has now become the first-choice treatment of chronic myelogenous leukemia especially when the diagnosis is made in the early stage of the disease and the patient has no compatible bone marrow donor.

IFN-α is effective against multiple myeloma. Objective responses have been obtained in 15–20% of previously treated patients, and a higher response rate in patients without previous treatment. However, the response rate of multiple myeloma to conventional chemotherapy is greater. Therefore, IFN-α is now used as an adjunct in the treatment of multiple myeloma to increase the response rate to chemotherapy by adding IFN-α to a conventional regimen [5], or to prolong the response duration by administering IFN-α as the maintenance therapy following induction therapy with combined chemotherapeutic agents [6].

A similar combination of IFN-α with cytotoxic chemotherapy was reported to prolong the time to treatment failure, and the duration of complete response in patients with clinically aggressive, low-grade and certain histological variants of intermediate-grade non-Hodgkin's lymphoma [7]. Combining IFN with conventional chemotherapy is now becoming the principal regimen for the treatment of multiple myeloma and non-Hodgkin's lymphoma.

For the treatment of solid tumors with IFN, malignant melanoma, metastatic renal cell carcinoma and AIDS-related Kaposi's sarcoma are the main malignancies for which IFN efficacy has been clinically documented. Although the response rates of malignant melanoma and metastatic renal cell carcinoma to IFN-α are as low as 10–20%, these advanced tumors are not responsive to conventional chemotherapy. An objective response rate by metastatic renal cell carcinoma of up to 20% was demonstrated in a phase II study of high-dose IFN-γ [8].

The combination of IFN-α with interleukin-2 (IL-2) resulted in an encouraging effect on renal cell carcinoma and malignant melanoma. Increasing the dose of both IFN-α and IL-2 induced a higher response rate, with maximum rates of 38 and 43%, respectively [9]. These values were apparently higher than those obtained by each cytokine alone. Similar efficacy of this combination on metastatic renal cell carcinoma has been reported by a German group [10]. It is therefore recommended that patients with metastatic renal cell carcinoma and malignant melanoma are treated by this combination of cytokines.

Other solid tumors against which IFNs have a significant effect are superficial bladder cancer, ovarian cancer and primary brain tumor (IFN-β). Intraperitoneal administration of IFN-α has also been effective against microscopic residual ovarian cancer [11].

The fluorinated pyrimidine, fluorouracil (5-FU), is the principal chemotherapeutic agent for disseminated colorectal cancer, although the response rate is low. Addition of IFN-α to 5-FU treatment was reported to increase the response rate to chemotherapy by this tumor [12]. In vitro studies demonstrated that the cytotoxicity to several cancer cell lines was the highest when 5-FU was combined with leucovorin and IFN-α [13].

IFN-γ has demonstrated activity against renal cell carcinoma, melanoma, mycosis fungoides, chronic myelogenous leukemia and ovarian cancer. Since IFN-γ reacts with a different cell surface receptor than IFN-α and IFN-β, there will be no cross-resistance. It may be possible to use IFN-γ in combination with IFN-α or IFN-β to potentiate the antitumor activity of IFNs. These clinical questions should be clarified through continuing clinical studies on IFNs.

**Interleukin-2**

IL-2 stimulates the growth of certain killer cells which are able to recognize and destroy tumor cells without damaging normal cells. These killer cells include the lymphokine-activated killer (LAK) cells, natural killer cells, cytotoxic T lymphocytes and tumor-infiltrating lymphocytes (TIL). Multiplication of these killer cells can be stimulated by IL-2 both in vitro and in vivo. This activity of IL-2 has been used for cancer treatment both alone and in combination with patients' lymphocytes harvested and grown in culture with IL-2 to induce LAK cells.

Clinical use of IL-2 for cancer treatment was initiated in 1985 by Rosenberg et al. [14]. Their studies were confirmed by other groups and the progress report on their original patients indicated 8 complete responses and 14 partial responses among 106 patients treated with IL-2 plus LAK cells. Complete responses were noted in patients with renal cell carcinoma, melanoma, colorectal cancer and non-Hodgkin's lymphoma. Renal cell carcinoma and malignant melanoma were the main targets of this adoptive immunotherapy, and response rates were 33 and 23%, respectively [15]. Adoptive immunotherapy using patients' cultured lymphocytes, however, is too expensive and time-consuming, with a very low cost: performance ratio, and routine clinical use of this therapy is not yet possible. Administration of IL-2 alone either by bolus or constant intravenous infusion has been the routine administration route for this cytokine. IL-2 was approved by the Food and Drug Administration (FDA) in the USA for renal cell carcinoma and malignant melanoma, while Ko-

**Table 1.** Hematopoietic growth factors and their primary effector cells

| Growth factor | | Effector cells |
|---|---|---|
| Granulocyte colony-stimulating factor | G-CSF | neutrophil |
| Granulocyte-macrophage colony-stimulating factor | GM-CSF | eosinophil, neutrophil, monocyte, macrophage |
| Macrophage colony-stimulating factor | M-CSF | monocyte, macrophage |
| Interleukin-3 | IL-3, multi-CSF | basophil, macrophage, megakaryocyte, red blood cell |
| Erythropoietin | EPO | red blood cell |

seisho of Japan approved the use of IL-2 only for malignant hemangioendothelioma [16].

Toxicity of IL-2 is a major problem. In addition to a flu-like syndrome which is common to most immunotherapy products, IL-2 induces characteristic hemodynamic abnormalities. Hypotension, body weight gain, accumulation of fluid in pleural as well as in peritoneal cavities are the main signs of the hypodynamic abnormality induced by IL-2. To avoid IL-2 toxicity, low-dose IL-2 was combined with cyclophosphamide [17] or dacarbazine [18] for the treatment of malignant melanoma. The response rate of this therapy was significantly higher than other IL-2-alone therapies. During the combination treatment with IL-2 and cyclophosphamide, induction of LAK cell activation was observed in all responding patients, and none of the patients without LAK activation had a remission [17].

Another approach to reduce the toxicity of IL-2 and to improve efficacy is to use TIL rather than LAK cells to induce cytotoxic cells by IL-2. Results of early clinical studies were encouraging [19]. However, use of TIL is limited, with difficulties in obtaining TIL from tumors, and the necessity for 4–5 weeks to grow TIL to therapeutic quantities. This time period is unacceptably long in the care of patients with advanced cancer.

IL-2 has also been administered intracavitarily as a palliative therapy for neoplastic effusions due to solid tumors. An objective response was achieved in 10/14 (71%) patients without significant toxicity and with a median duration of 4 months [20].

Murine bone marrow cells activated with IL-2 in vitro demonstrated potent graft-versus-leukemia (GVL) and anticytomegalovirus effects in an experimental syngenic bone marrow transplantation setting followed by IL-2 therapy. Human bone marrow cells which were treated with IL-2 in vitro purged leukemic cells without loss of progenitor cell activity [21]. It is, therefore, expected that IL-2 will be used in autologous as well as allogenic bone marrow transplantation to increase the GVL effect and to abolish graft-versus-host disease.

## Hematopoietic Growth Factors

The first hematopoietic factor which was produced by recombinant technology and became clinically available was erythropoietin (EPO). Although EPO was approved only for anemia associated with renal failure, this hematopoietic growth factor is effective for various kinds of anemia including that associated with malignancy. For an unknown reason, EPO levels are inappropriately low in cancer-associated anemia, and EPO deficiency may contribute to the development of anemia in cancer patients [22]. EPO administration to patients with multiple myeloma and low-grade non-Hodgkin's lymphoma induced a significant increase in hemoglobin levels leading to an eventual correction of the anemia [23, 24]. EPO was also effective for the chemotherapy-induced anemia of cancer patients [25]. Administration of EPO, therefore, should be tried in cancer patients with associated refractory anemia which needs red cell transfusions.

Colony-stimulating factors (CSFs) are classified as multi-CSF (IL-3), granulocyte-macrophage (GM-CSF), macrophage (M-CSF) and granulocyte (G-CSF) according to the maturational stages of the main targeted hematopoietic precursor cells and the kinds of effector cells (table 1). Among these CSFs, recombinant GM-CSF and recombinant G-CSF are approved for clinical use in patients with various kinds of neutropenia. Native M-CSF partially purified from human urine is approved in

Japan for neutropenias. M-CSF was demonstrated to stimulate the production of GM-CSF and G-CSF by monocytes-macrophages [26].

Recombinant CSFs vary in their degree of glycosylation depending on the type of host cells used for their production. However, the recombinant products appear to be biologically as well as clinically equivalent to the native glycosylated CSFs.

Clinical trials of GM-CSF and G-CSF performed on cancer patients with associated chemotherapy-induced neutropenia clearly demonstrated that neutropenia was significantly less severe and shorter in the cycles with CSFs as compared with those without [27–32]. The frequency of infectious complications was significantly reduced following administration of CSFs, and patients needed fewer days of antibiotic treatment. Dose intensification of cytotoxic drugs was also possible using CSFs. Although not yet clearly documented, it is believed that the administration of CSFs will increase remission duration after cytotoxic treatment, and prolong the survival of cancer patients. G-CSF has higher specificity in its action on neutrophils than GM-CSF, and has fewer adverse effects than GM-CSF. It is, therefore, much more useful than GM-CSF in the clinical situation in which only the stimulation of the production and function of neutrophils is required.

CSFs are effective in accelerating recovery from neutropenia after autologous as well as allogenic bone marrow transplantation. GM-CSF and G-CSF significantly reduced the number of days required for granulocyte recovery after bone marrow transplantation. The number of febrile days and days in the clean room were also significantly reduced [28, 33–37].

The total cost of cancer chemotherapy and bone marrow transplantation can be reduced using CSFs, as a result of the reduced frequency of administration of antimicrobial drugs and a shorter stay in hospital.

In vivo administration of GM-CSF and G-CSF induces an increased production of hematopoietic stem cells in the bone marrow, and an increased release of hematopoietic stem cells into the circulation. This effect of CSFs can be used for the efficient collection of bone marrow cells from the donor for bone marrow transplantation as well as for the peripheral blood stem cell harvest for transplantation, which has to be studied as an alternative or an adjunct to bone marrow transplantation [37, 38].

Stem cell factor (SCF), a hematopoietic growth factor identified as a ligand to the c-*kit* receptor has been demonstrated to stimulate the production of hematopoietic stem cells in vitro and in vivo [39]. It induced an increase in peripheral blood stem cells in baboons [40]. Combined administration of CSFs and SCF may be most effective in increasing the number of peripheral blood stem cells.

A combination of hematopoietic growth factors is also used to increase in vitro the clonogenic colony-forming cells from human peripheral blood CD34+ stem cells. A mixture of G-CSF, GM-CSF, M-CSF, IL-1, IL-3, IL-6 and SCF was most effective in increasing the number of colony-forming cells [41]. It is expected that by combining hematopoietic growth factors in vivo and in vitro, we can reduce the number of bone marrow cells taken from the donor for bone marrow transplantation to the extent that general anesthesia will not be needed, or we can use peripheral blood stem cell transplantation as an alternative to bone marrow transplantation.

Thrombocytopenia occurs very often after cytotoxic chemotherapy. No specific hematopoietic growth factor has been identified despite a long history of research to identify the factor termed thrombopoietin. Animal experiments and preliminary clinical trials have shown that IL-1, IL-3, IL-6 and IL-11 can increase peripheral blood thrombocytes and accelerate the recovery from chemotherapy-induced thrombocytopenia [42–44].

The thrombopoietic effect of these cytokines, however, was not as strong as we would expect for a specific thrombopoietin. Moreover, all these ILs have fairly strong adverse effects. We have to devise a good combination of these ILs or make new IL mutants which have fewer side effects and much more potent thrombopoietic activity if we want to use these cytokines clinically as the thrombopoietic growth factor.

Transplantation of peripheral blood stem cells released from bone marrow after stimulation with G-CSF demonstrated an acceleration of the rate of recovery from thrombocytopenia after cytotoxic chemotherapy [38].

To protect the hematopoietic stem cells from injury during the administration of cytotoxic drugs, the recombinant stem cell inhibitor (SCI), macrophage inflammatory protein 1, was injected into mice receiving cytosine arabinoside. Injection of SCI induced a marked and dose-dependent decrease of immature hematopoietic stem cells in S phase in the bone marrow. The mice injected with SCI showed a significant improvement in the kinetics of neutrophil recovery [45].

CSFs have been demonstrated mainly by in vitro studies or by animal experiments to have cytotoxic activity against cancer cells through the stimulation of monocytes-macrophages or neutrophils. Several cytotoxic cytokines such as IFNs and tumor necrosis factor (TNF) are produced by these cells after stimulation with CSFs. Antibody-dependent cytotoxicity exerted by these cells is also enhanced after stimulation with CSFs. However, there have been no clinical studies indicating the anticancer activity of CSFs.

## Cytokines and Gene Therapy

The first gene therapy using a cytokine was initiated by Rosenberg and his group in 1991. They transduced TIL from malignant melanoma patients with human TNF cDNA. These TIL expressing TNF were expected to have potent cytotoxic activity against melanoma cells when used for adoptive immunotherapy. However, there has been no report on the results of this immunotherapy. Their group obtained further approval from the recombinant-DNA advisory committee of the NIH on a protocol of gene therapy for cancer. In that protocol they will transduce cancer cells with human TNF or IL-2 cDNA. TIL sensitized by transduced cancer cells will be used for adoptive immunotherapy of malignancies.

In many gene therapy protocols, transduced T lymphocytes and bone marrow or peripheral blood stem cells are used as the carriers of effective genes or as the in vivo marker. The long life of these cells is considered to be advantageous for these purposes. To transduce human cDNAs using a retroviral vector, the target cells should be cell cycling. For this purpose, IL-2 is used for T lymphocytes, and a combination of IL-3, IL-6 and SCF for stem cells. Many protocols for human gene therapy would not have been realized without the development of cytokines [46]. The availability of various cytokines has made a great contribution to the recent progress in gene therapy of human diseases including cancer.

## References


1 Quesda JR, Reuken J, Manning JT, Hersh EM, Gutterman JU: Alpha interferon for induction of remission in hairy cell leukemia. N Engl J Med 1984;310:15–18.
2 Smith JW I, Longs DL, Urba WJ, Clark JW, Watson T, Beveridge J, Colon KC, Sznol M, Creekmore SP, Alvord WG, Lawrence JB, Steis R: Prolonged, continuous treatment of hairy cell leukemia patients with recombinant interferon-α2a. Blood 1971;78:1664–1671.
3 Talpaz M, McCredie KB, Mavligit GM, Gutterman JU: Leukocyte interferon-induced myeloid cytoreduction in chronic myelogenous leukemia. Blood 1983;62:689–692.
4 Talpaz M, Kantarijian HM, McCredic KB, Trujillo JM, Keating MJ, Gutterman JU: Hematologic remission and cytogenetic improvement induced by recombinant human interferon alpha A in chronic myelogenous leukemia. N Engl J Med 1986;314:1065–1069.
5 Montuoro A, DeRosa L, DeBlasio A, Pacilli L, Petti N, De Laurenzi A: Alpha-2a-interferon/melphalan/prednisone versus melphalan/prednisone in previously untreated patients with multiple myeloma. Br J Haematol 1990;76:365–368.
6 Mandelli F, Avvisati G, Amadori S, Boccadoro M, Gernone A, Lauta VM, Marmont F, Petrucci MT, Tribalto M, Vegna ML, Dammacco F, Pileri A: Maintenance treatment with recombinant interferon alfa-2b in patients with multiple myeloma responding to conventional induction chemotherapy. N Engl J Med 1990;322:1430–1434.
7 Smalley RV, Anderson JW, Hawking MJ, Bhide V, O'Connell MJ, Oken MM, Borden EC: Interferon alfa combined with cytotoxic chemotherapy for patients with non-Hodgkin's lymphoma. N Engl J Med 1992;327:1336–1341.
8 Recombinant Human Interferon Gamma (S-6810) Research Group on Renal Cell Carcinoma: Phase II study of recombinant human interferon gamma (S-6810) on renal cell carcinoma: Summary of two collaborative studies. Cancer 1987;60:929–933.
9 Rosenberg SA, Lotze MT, Yang JC, Linehan WM, Seipp C, Calabro S, Karp SE, Sherry RM, Steinberg S, White DE: Combination therapy with interleukin-2 and alpha-interferon for the treatment of patients with advanced cancer. J Clin Oncol 1989;7:1863–1874.
10 Kirchner H, Körfer A, Palmer PA, Evers P, Riese WD, Knüver-Hopf J, Madman M, Goldman U, Franks CR, Poliwoda M, Atzpodien J: Subcutaneous interleukin-2 and interferon-α 2b in patients with metastatic renal cell cancer: The German outpatient experience. Mol Biother 1990;2:145–154.
11 Berck JS: Intraperitoneal immunotherapy for ovarian cancer with alpha interferon. Eur J Cancer 1992;20A:719–721.
12 Wadler S, Schwartz EL, Goldman M, Lyver A, Rader M, Zimmerman M, Itri L, Weinberg V, Wiernik PH: Fluorouracil and recombinant alfa-2a-interferon: An active regimen against advanced colorectal carcinoma. J Clin Oncol 1989;7:1769–1775.
13 Rastum YM: Rational basis for the metabolic modulation of 5-fluorouracil by leucovorin and interferon alfa. Br J Haematol 1991;19(suppl 1):52–55.
14 Rosenberg SA, Lotze MT, Mull LM, Lettman A, Chang AE, Ettinghausen SE, Matory YL, Skibber JM, Shiloni E, Vetto JT, Seipp CA, Simpson C, Reichert C: Observations on the systemic administration of autologous lymphokine-activated killer cells and recombinant interleukin-2 to patients with metastatic cancer. N Engl J Med 1985;313:1485–1492.
15 Rosenberg SA, Lotze MT, Muul LM, Chang AE, Avis FP, Leitman S, Linehan WM, Rosenberg CN, Lee RE, Rubin JT, Seip CA, Simpson CG, White DE: A progress report on the treatment of 157 patients with advanced cancer using lymphokine-activated killer cells and interleukin-2 or high-dose interleukin-2 alone. N Engl J Med 1987;316:889–897.
16 Masuzawa M, Higashi K, Nishioka K, Nishiyama S: Successful immunotherapy for malignant hemangioendothelioma using recombinant interleukin-2 (in Japanese). Jpn J Dermatol 1988;98:367–369.
17 Mitchell MS, Kempt RA, Harel W, Shau H, Boswell WD, Lind S, Bradley EC: Effectiveness and tolerability of low-dose cyclophosphamide and low-dose intravenous interleukin-2 in disseminated melanoma. J Clin Oncol 1988;6:409–424.
18 Flaherty L, Redman B, Chabot G, Martino S, Valdivieso M, Bradley E: Combination of dacarbazine and interleukin-2 in metastatic malignant melanoma (abstract). Proc Am Soc Clin Oncol 1988;7:254.

19 Rosenberg SA, Packard BS, Aebersold PM, Solomon D, Topalian SL, Toy ST, Simon P, Lotze MT, Yang JC, Seipp CA, Simpson C, Carter C, Bock S, Schwartzentruber D, Wei JP, White DE: Use of tumor-infiltrating lymphocytes and interleukin-2 in the immunotherapy of patients with metastatic melanoma. N Engl J Med 1988;319:1676–1680.
20 Lissoni P, Barni S, Ardizzoia A, Paolorossi F, Tisi E, Crispino S, Tancini G: Intracavitary administration of interleukin-2 as palliative therapy for neoplastic effusions. Tumori 1992; 78:118–120.
21 Charak BS, Chondhary GD, Tefft M, Mazumder A: Interleukin-2 in bone marrow transplantation: Preclinical studies. Bone Marrow Transplant 1992;10:103–111.
22 Miller CB, Jones RJ, Piantadosi S, Abeloff MD, Spivak JL: Decreased erythropoietin response in patients with the anemia of cancer. N Engl J Med 1990;322:1684–1692.
23 Ludwig M, Fritz E, Kotzmann H, Hocker P, Gisslinger H, Barnas U: Erythropoietin treatment of anemia associated with multiple myeloma. N Engl J Med 1990;322:1693–1699.
24 Oster W, Herrmann F, Gamm H, Zeile G, Lindermann A, Muller G, Brune T, Kaemer HP, Mertelsmann R: Erythropoietin for the treatment of anemia of malignancy associated with neoplastic bone marrow infiltration. J Clin Oncol 1990;8:956–962.
25 Oster W, Mertelsmann R: Erythropoietin for the treatment of patients with anemia of malignancy; in Mertelsmann R, Hermann F (eds): Hematopoietic Growth Factors in Clinical Applications. New York, Marcel Dekker, 1990, pp 141–148.
26 Motoyoshi K, Yoshida K, Hatake K, Saito M, Miura Y, Yanai N, Yamada M, Kawashima T, Wong GG, Temple PA, Leary AC, Witek-Giamotti JS, Fujisawa M, Yuo A, Okabe T, Takaku F: Recombinant and native human urinary colony-stimulating factor directly augments granulocyte and granulocyte-macrophage colony-stimulating factor production of human peripheral blood monocytes. Exp Hematol 1989; 17:68–71.
27 Antman KS, Griffin JD, Elias A, Socinski MA, Ryan L, Lannistra SA, Oette D, Whitley M, Frei E III, Schnipper LE: Effect of human granulocyte-macrophage colony-stimulating factor on chemotherapy-induced myelosuppression. N Engl J Med 1988;319:593–598.
28 Schulz G, Frisch J, Greifenberg B, Nicolay U, Oster W: New therapeutic modalities for the clinical use of rhGM-CSF in patients with malignancies. Am J Clin Oncol 1991;14(suppl 1): 19–26.
29 Morstyn G, Campbell L, Souza LM, Alton NK, Keech J, Green M, Sheridan W, Metcalf D: Effect of granulocyte colony stimulating factor on neutropenia induced by cytotoxic chemotherapy. Lancet 1988;i:667–672.
30 Gabrilove JL, Jakubowski A, Scher H, Sternberg C, Wong G, Grous J, Yogoda A, Faui K, Moore MAS, Clarkson B, Oetigen HF, Alton K, Welte K, Souza LM: Effect of granulocyte colony-stimulating factor on neutropenia and associated morbidity due to chemotherapy for transitional-cell carcinoma of the urothelium. N Engl J Med 1988;318:1414–1422.
31 Bronchud MM, Howell A, Crowther D, Hopwood P, Souza LM, Dexter TM: The use of granulocyte colony-stimulating factor to increase the intensity of treatment with doxorubicin in patients with advanced breast and ovarian cancer. Br J Cancer 1989;60:121–125.
32 Takaku F: Clinical use of human granulocyte colony stimulating factor; in Clark SC, Golde DW (eds): Hematopoiesis. New York, Alan R Liss, 1990, pp 217–227.
33 Brandt SJ, Peters WP, Atwater SK, Kurtzberg J, Borowitz MJ, Jones RB, Shpall EJ, Bast RC Jr, Gilbert CJ, Oette DH: Effect of recombinant human granulocyte-macrophage colony stimulating factor on hematopoietic reconstitution after high-dose chemotherapy and autologous bone marrow transplantation. N Engl J Med 1988;318:869–876.
34 Neumaniatis J, Singer JW, Buckner D, Hill R, Storb R, Thomas ED, Appelbaum FR: Use of recombinant human granulocyte-macrophage colony-stimulating factor in autologous marrow transplantation for lymphoid malignancies. Blood 1988;72:834–836.
35 Taylor K, Jagannath S, Spitzer G, Spinolo JA, Tucker SL, Fogel B, Cabanillas FF, Magemeister EB, Souza LM: Recombinant human granulocyte colony-stimulating factor hastens granulocyte recovery after high-dose chemotherapy and autologous bone marrow transplantation in Hodgkin's disease. J Clin Oncol 1989;7: 1791–1799.
36 Asano S, Masaoka T, Takaku F: Beneficial effect of recombinant human glycosylated granulocyte colony-stimulating factor in marrow transplanted patients: Results of multicenter phase II-III studies. Transplant Proc 1991;23:1701–1703.
37 Haas R, Mo AD, Bredthauer U, Cayeux S, Egerer G, Knauf W, Hunstein W: Successful autologous transplantation of blood stem cells mobilized with recombinant human GM-CSF. Exp Hematol 1990;18:94–98.
38 Sheridan WP, Begley CG, Jutter CA, Szer J, To LB, Maher D, McGrath KM, Morstyn G, Fox RM: Effect of peripheral-blood progenitor cells mobilized by filgrastim(G-CSF) on platelet recovery after high-dose chemotherapy. Lancet 1992;399:640–644.
39 Brandt J, Briddell RA, Srour EF, Leemhuis TB, Hoffman R: Role of c-*kit* ligand in the expansion of human hematopoietic progenitor cells. Blood 1992;79:634–641.
40 Andrews RG, Bensinger WI, Knitter GH, Bartelmez SH, Longin K, Bernstein ID, Appelbaum FR, Zsebo KM: The ligand for c-*kit*, stem cell factor(SCF), stimulates the circulation of cells that engraft lethally irradiated baboons. Blood 1992;80:2715–2720.
41 Haylock DN, To LB, Dowse TL, Juttner CA, Simmons PJ: Ex vivo expansion and maturation of peripheral blood CD34 cells into the myeloid lineage. Blood 1992;80:1405–1412.
42 Smith JW, Longo D, Alvord W, Janik J, Shanfran W, Gause B, Curti B, Sznol M, Steis R, Miller L, Fenton R, Creekmore S, Holmlund J, Feim S, Shimize M, Oppenheim J, Hursey J, Houck M, Rubi WJ: Thrombopoietic effects of IL-1 alpha in combination with high dose carboplatin. Proc Am Soc Clin Oncol 1992;11: 820a.
43 Stahl CP, Winton EF, Monroe MC, Haff E, Holman RC, Myers L, Liehl E, Evatt BL: Differential effect of sequential, simultaneous and single agent interleukin-3 and granulocyte-macrophage colony-stimulating factor on megakaryocyte maturation and platelet response in primates. Blood 1992;80:2479–2485.
44 Asano S, Okano A, Ozawa K, Nakahata T, Ishibashi T, Koike K, Kimura H, Tanioka Y, Shibuya A, Hirano T, Kishimoto T, Takaku F, Akiyama Y: In vivo effects of recombinant human interleukin-6 in primates: Stimulated production of platelets. Blood 1990;75:1602–1605.
45 Dunlop DJ, Wright EG, Lorimore S, Graham GJ, Holyoake T, Kerr DJ, Wolpe SD, Pragnell IB: Demonstration of stem cell inhibition and myeloprotective effect of SCI/rhMIPI in vivo. Blood 1992;79:2221–2225.
46 Miller AD: Human gene therapy comes of age. Nature 1992;357:455–460.

Oncology 1994;51:129–136

*Sanjiv S. Agarwala*
*John M. Kirkwood*

Division of Medical Oncology,
Pittsburgh Cancer Institute,
University of Pittsburgh Medical Center,
Pittsburgh, Pa., USA

# Interferons in the Therapy of Solid Tumors

**Key Words**
Interferons
Therapy
Tumors
Melanoma
Review
Systemic
Immunotherapy
Chemotherapy

**Abstract**
Interferons, a group of naturally occurring proteins, possess potent immunological effects. The availability of large amounts of purified interferon through recombinant DNA technology has led to the testing of these agents against a number of tumor types. Interferon-α has been the most widely studied. The most encouraging results have been observed in the treatment of melanoma among nonhematological neoplasms, and in the locoregional treatment of other tumor types. It is hoped that further research into the use of the interferons, both singly and in combination with chemotherapy and other immunological agents, will lead to a better elucidation of their therapeutic role against cancer. In this article, the use of interferons in the treatment of solid tumors is reviewed.

## Introduction

The interferons (IFNs) are a group of naturally occurring proteins that are produced in response to viral, antigenic or mitogenic stimuli. Since their discovery in 1957, they have been found to have potent effects on immune function and tumor biology, in addition to their antiviral actions. IFNs are broadly divided into two classes: type I (IFN-α and IFN-β) and type II (IFN-γ). Type I IFNs may be produced by all human cells and share a range of biological effects. The physiologic stimuli for their production are diverse and include infectious agents and their component nucleic acids. In contrast, type II IFNs are produced only by T lymphocytes and natural killer (NK) cells and possess actions discrete from type I IFNs mediated through a separate receptor. The physiologic stimulus for IFN-γ appears to be antigen/mitogen stimulation and interleukin-2 (IL-2).

The advent of recombinant DNA technology and the consequent availability of large amounts of purified IFNs have led to the broad examination of these agents against various tumors. IFN-α has been the most extensively studied agent, although clinical data regarding IFN-γ are accumulating rapidly. Here we review the current role of IFNs in the therapy of solid tumors.

## Cutaneous Melanoma

*Clinical Antitumor Efficacy*

IFN-α was first investigated in large multicenter trials in the United States as a therapeutic modality for melanoma by the American Cancer Society Interferon Working Group beginning in 1978. More than twelve phase II trials have now been fully published, documenting the antitumor activity of systemically administered recombinant IFNs in melanoma [1–4]. Aggregate response rates of approximately 16%, with complete responses of 6% have been reported.

Clinical and other prognostic factors that may predict responsiveness to IFN have been sought. Patients with only cutaneous, soft-tissue, and pulmonary disease of low

John M. Kirkwood, MD
Division of Medical Oncology, Pittsburgh Cancer Institute
University of Pittsburgh Medical Center
3459 Fifth Avenue, 7 Main North
Pittsburgh, PA 15213-2592 (USA)


0030–2414/94/0512–0129
$5.00/0

bulk have been reported to be most likely to benefit from IFN, but visceral disease responses have also been reported [1, 5]. The prognostic effect of prior treatment has been examined in two large experiences at the Mayo Clinic [6] and M.D. Anderson Cancer Center [1], revealing no adverse impact of prior chemotherapy, hormonal therapy, or radiation therapy upon the likelihood of response to IFN-α2a. Patients with minimal disease, particularly involving lymph node and cutaneous sites, tend to demonstrate higher response rates.

Of note is the time required to achieve response in these studies, with median intervals to complete response of 3 months, and responses observed after as long as 6 months of therapy [1, 3]. A number of phase II trials have consequently required treatment for a minimum of 3 months for response evaluability, although the majority of patients show some evidence of response by the end of the first month.

Complete responses obtained in the earliest series have been disease-free for as long as 7 years, and a recent summary of long-term responders has shown no distinguishing features of the disease in these patients that might allow prediction of response [3, 5]. Whether or not maintenance therapy enhances the durability of complete response has not been established. The median duration of partial responses observed with IFN-α2 is 4 months.

Review of the treatment protocols utilizing IFN-α suggests that the best results have been obtained with uninterrupted schedules, regardless of the route of administration, at a dose of between $10 \times 10^6$ U/m$^2$ daily and $50 \times 10^6$ U/m$^2$ every other day [3, 6]. The only studies of IFN-α2 in which there were markedly reduced response rates (no response in 15 subjects) [7] involved intermittent treatment with IFN-α2a given 5 days out of every 14, or IFN-α2b given 5 days out of every 21 [5].

Anti-IFN antibodies have been detected in up to 5% of patients after 2–6 months of therapy [2], but it is uncertain whether this impacts on therapeutic effect. Initial therapy with intravenous (i.v.), as opposed to subcutaneous (s.c.) or intramuscular (i.m.), routes, and continuous, as opposed to interrupted schedules, may reduce the immunogenicity of recombinant IFNs.

*Regional Therapy with IFN-α*

Intralesional administration of IFN-α has been examined by a number of investigators. When administered intralesionally or perilesionally at a dose of $6 \times 10^6$–$10 \times 10^6$ U twice or three times weekly, in a series of 51 patients, 3 complete responses and 6 partial responses were noted, some in lesions remote from the sites of IFN administration, such as the lung [8].

*Systemic Combination Therapy of Melanoma with IFN-α*

IFN-α has been combined with a variety of other agents in an attempt to enhance its immunomodulatory, differentiating, or cytotoxic effects. These include cimetidine, indomethacin, low-dose cyclophosphamide, DFMO (eflornithine), and dacarbazine (DTIC).

The basis for the use of cimetidine and low-dose cyclophosphamide derives from experimental murine and in vitro human studies which suggest a role of suppressor T lymphocytes in the progression of cancer, and the discovery of H-2 histamine receptors expressed by suppressor T lymphocytes. An early trial reported a relatively high response rate of 30% [9]; however, other attempts to corroborate the initial positive trials have not shown any enhancement of response [10]. Two trials combining IFN-α with DFMO, an irreversible inhibitor of ornithine decarboxylase, have shown no evidence for enhanced antitumor efficacy [11, 12].

The rationale for administration of IFN-α in combination with dacarbazine has been to combine two of the most active single agents available for systemic therapy of melanoma. Two large trials have tested somewhat different dose combinations with contradictory results. An uncontrolled Australian trial carried out in 44 patients utilizing IFN-α2a with dacarbazine escalated to tolerance showed complete responses in 6 patients and partial responses in an additional 7 (an overall response rate of 30%) [13]. A randomized controlled trial of IFN-α2b administered alone versus dacarbazine versus the combination of the two agents has been preliminarily reported to yield virtually identical response rates in the combined treatment arm and the dacarbazine-only arm [14, 15]. The true role of the combination of IFNs and dacarbazine in the treatment of metastatic melanoma thus awaits definitive evaluation. An Eastern Cooperative Oncology Group (ECOG) study (EST 3690) is currently testing dacarbazine with or without IFN with or without tamoxifen in a $2 \times 2$ design, that ought to unequivocally establish the presence or absence of synergism with these agents.

IFN has been combined with other agents in more limited clinical trials including cisplatin [16], low-dose cyclophosphamide as an immunomodulator [17], and indomethacin [18], with no major benefit from any combination thus far.

*Systemic IFN-γ*

Several trials of IFN-γ administered alone, and a number of trials exploring combinations of IFN-γ with other biologicals have been reported [19–21]. The role of this agent in the therapy of melanoma at this point is still undefined. Phase I-II dose-seeking studies have been coordinated through cooperative groups in the US and Europe. To date, very little antitumor activity has been noted, either in single-institution or cooperative group trials [22].

*Adjuvant Applications of the IFNs*

Various trials exploring this issue are nearing analysis and/or completion [23]. The WHO Melanoma Programme is conducting a controlled trial of chronic low-dose IFN-α (3 $\times 10^6$ U/m$^2$ s.c. three times a week for 2–3 years following resection of regional lymph node metastases). The ECOG has initiated a three-arm trial of high dosages of IFN-α2b for 1 year versus low dosages of IFN-α2b for at least 2 years, versus control (EST 1690). This trial is more than half-completed, but will not be analyzed until 1994.

## Renal Cell Carcinoma

Renal cell carcinoma (RCC) afflicts approximately 23,000 people annually in the United States resulting in 10,000 deaths [24]. No effective chemotherapy exists for this tumor: vinblastine, the most effective single agent, produces a response rate of less than 15% [25]. The IFNs have been extensively studied as therapy for this tumor both as single agents and in combination with other cytotoxic and humoral modalities.

More than 1,000 patients with RCC have been treated with recombinant-DNA-produced IFNs as single agents, achieving an overall response rate of 10–15% [26, 27]. Of these responses, only 2% have been complete. Earlier trials using leukocyte or lymphoblastoid IFN were reported to induce higher response rates of up to 20%, possibly due to the presence of other immunomodulators in these preparations. There is no convincing evidence that any one particular IFN preparation is superior to any other. Current reports in the literature suggest that higher doses may be associated with superior response rates at the expense of greater toxicity, although some of the trials using low doses were of short duration, and may have failed to detect responses to IFN which may occur in RCC as late as 6 months after treatment. Trials associated with higher response rates were conducted at dosages of between 5 $\times 10^6$ and 10 $\times 10^6$ U daily.

No obvious prognostic features separating responders from nonresponders have been identified, with the exception of pulmonary metastatic disease which displays the greatest response of up to 30%. The role of nephrectomy is controversial, but a recent report suggests an improved response to IFN-α2a in patients who underwent nephrectomy within the 12 months preceding the onset of therapy [28]. Patients with favorable performance status seem to do better, but such patients are also likely to tolerate therapy at maximum dose and to have a lower tumor burden.

*IFNs in Combination with Other Biologicals*

The concept of combined usage of biological therapies is attractive because of in vitro data indicating synergistic antitumor effects of a number of cytokines. IFNs may augment the immune response by inducing major histocompatibility (MHC) antigens, and enhanced effector cell function, including T cell and NK cell activity, and may thus be logically predicted to potentiate the response to other lymphokines, including IL-2.

Numerous trials utilizing combination IFN and IL-2 have been reported [29, 30]. The treatment appears to be well tolerated and can be administered in the outpatient setting or even at home. The actual role of this combination, however, awaits definition through larger randomized trials.

The knowledge that IFN-α and IFN-γ have different receptors, and the observation that IFN-γ can modulate the IFN-α receptor has led to trials with combination therapy with these two preparations. In general, response rates have not been superior to either agent alone except for one study which showed response rates of 32% using sequential as opposed to simultaneous therapy [31]. This may be due to the limitations imposed by the overlapping toxicity from concurrent administration of IFN-α and IFN-γ. The role of sequential administration of these two agents is currently being tested in cooperative group trials (EST 6890).

In vitro data suggesting a synergy between IFN and tumor necrosis factor has led to attempts to combine these two agents clinically [32].

*IFN in Combination with Chemotherapy*

Vinblastine, the most effective chemotherapeutic agent for RCC, has been the focus of chemotherapy-IFN combinations. Synergism between these two agents has been demonstrated in vitro [33]. Response rates to treatment of human RCC with the combination have only been marginally better than those of either agent alone [34, 35]. Other agents which have been tried include doxorubicin [26] and cyclophosphamide [17], but without improved clinical efficacy.

## Breast Carcinoma

Despite major therapeutic advances in the management of breast cancer, the overall prognosis for patient with metastatic disease remains poor and no change in survival can be demonstrated over the past 20 years. Intensive chemotherapy with or without autologous bone marrow or hematopoietic growth factor support has improved the outlook in terms of response rates, but the impact of this therapy upon breast cancer has yet to be established, and newer treatment modilities are clearly needed. Unfortunately, trials with recombinant IFNs in breast cancer have been disappointing [36, 37] with an overall response rate of under 10%. Again, the earliest trials of leukocyte buffy coat IFN-α were reported to yield higher response rates, implying that other cytokines present as impurities may have had a role in the therapeutic response. Subsequent negative trials, however, used heavily pretreated patients with refractory and drug-resistant disease.

A number of reports have indicated that exposure of breast cancer cell lines to IFN-α increase estrogen receptors and sensitivity to tamoxifen [38, 39]. As an extension of this, clinical trials using combinations of tamoxifen and IFN have been carried out in patients with metastatic disease [40–42], without significant impact upon efficacy. In the adjuvant setting, a randomized study comparing the combination of cyclophosphamide and doxorubicin with or without IFN-α showed no benefit from the combination [43].

Local instillation of IFN into metastatic skin lesions [44] or intrapleurally in patients with pleural carcinomatosis [45] has produced more encouraging results, as noted with locoregional therapy of other tumor types.

Overall, IFNs have not achieved a significant place in the management of breast cancer, either in the adjuvant setting, or in patients with metastatic disease.

## Ovarian Cancer

IFN has been shown to exhibit in vitro synergism with cisplatin against ovarian cancer cell lines [46]. Modulation of MHC and tumor-associated antigens has also been demonstrated following exposure of cells to IFN-α [47]. Trials for the treatment of ovarian cancer using IFNs have been performed using both the parenteral and intraperitoneal (i.p.) routes of administration.

Systemically administered IFN has produced response rates of between 10–15% [48, 49]. A combination of lymphoblastoid IFN administered along with cyclophosphamide, doxorubicin and cisplatin proved unacceptably toxic [50].

IFN has been used i.p. to eradicate minimal residual disease following surgery. A pathologically confirmed complete response rate at second-look laparotomy of 45% was observed in one trial, where response was inversely related to maximum tumor diameter [51]. Another trial that combined i.p. IFN with cisplatin reported a response rate of 50% [52]. Systemic absorption and subsequent toxicity occurs with i.p. administration, but peritoneal fluid-to-serum peak concentration ratios of between 30 and 1,000 have been attained. Residual tumors >5 mm tend not to respond, indicating tumor bulk as a major prognostic factor. A recently reported cooperative group study failed to corroborate these earlier impressive results, and reported a response rate of only 5% in 18 patients using the same therapeutic strategy. Most of their study group was initially refractory to platinum [53]. A 43% response rate has been observed with combined IFN-α and carboplatinum [54]. Further trials are needed to define the role of i.p. IFN particularly in combination with cisplatin and its analogs.

IFN-α has also been used i.p. in the management of patients with recurrent malignant ascites due to ovarian cancer, with favorable results [55, 56]. Combinations of IFN and cisplatin by the i.p. route appear to be more effective than either agent alone [56].

## Colorectal Carcinoma

Current therapy for advanced colorectal carcinoma using fluorouracil (5-FU), the most active agent, produces response rates of less than 20% and does not influence patient survival. IFN, given alone, has been shown to be devoid of antitumor activity. However, IFN may modulate the activity of 5-FU: laboratory data suggest a synergistic cytotoxic response of these two agents against certain colon cancer cell lines [57]. Various mechanisms have been proposed to explain this synergism, including enhanced inhibition of thymidylate synthetase (TS) and increased accumulation of FdUMP, the active metabolite of 5-FU [58]. Inhibition of TS production by tumor cells may also play a role. A recent pharmacokinetic study of the effects of a combination of 5-FU and IFN showed that serum levels of 5-FU rose 16-fold when IFN was administered during 5-FU infusion [59].

Three major clinical trials of 5-FU with IFN-α have been published [60–62]. All three trials used a loading dose of continuous infusion 5-FU for 5 days followed by weekly 5-FU along with s.c. IFN-α, 9 × $10^6$ U three times a week. A total of 112 patients were treated, producing response rates of between 26 and 63%. Major toxicities included diarrhea, mucositis, leukopenia and neurotoxicity. These encouranging results have led to the examination of this regimen against of range of gastrointestinal malignancies in ongoing trials.

It is well established that the action of 5-FU against colon cancer can be modulated by folinic acid (FA), producing improved clinical efficacy, and that this modulation occurs through a mechanism distinct from that of IFN-α. Combined treatment with 5-FU, FA and IFN-α may thus produce an additive effect. A number of recent studies testing this hypothesis have, however, failed to show any benefit over the established 5-FU/FA regime [63, 64].

## Bladder Cancer

Carcinoma of the bladder accounts for about 2% of all malignant tumors and an estimated 52,300 new cases will occur in 1993 [24]. Nearly 90% appear to be localized at the time of diagnosis, but more than 75% will recur. IFNs have been investigated mainly as intravesical therapy for the management of carcinoma in situ (CIS) or to decrease recurrence rates from superficial cancer.

Bladder cancer is one of the few solid tumors which exhibits a definite response to immunotherapy. The agent most widely used to date and against which newer therapies are to be judged is bacillus Calmette-Guérin (BCG) which has produced complete response rates of up to 70% [65]. Other agents used intravesically include mitomycin, thio-TEPA and doxorubicin. Their use has been limited by systemic absorption leading to myelosuppression and chemical cystitis.

Recent studies with IFN-α2b have demonstrated significant activity against CIS with greater response rates at a dosage of 100 × $10^6$ versus 10 × $10^6$ (43 vs. 5% complete response) [66].

Safety and tolerance were reported to be excellent with a marked lack of local irritative toxicity. Encapsulation of IFN-α within liposomes that may selectively target bladder cancer cells may further augment its antiproliferative activity [67].

IFN-α has also been used in an attempt to decrease the rate of local recurrence of superficial bladder cancer given on a daily to a weekly schedule. Encouraging results have been reported by a number of investigators [68–70]; once again, the higher dose of IFN seemed to be more effective. An attempt has also been made to combine IFN-α2b with epirubicin for the same purpose [71]. Overall, results equal to BCG and superior to intravesical chemotherapy have been obtained with significantly less toxicity.

Systemic IFN used as treatment for metastatic disease has been less promising. However, a recent study from the National Cancer Institute that combined 5-FU and IFN-α2a, suggested synergy between these two agents in a small series of patients with advanced metastatic and chemotherapy-refractory disease, and warrants further study [72].

IFN-γ has been demonstrated to inhibit the growth of various bladder carcinoma cell lines [73, 74], suggesting that this agent may be of promise, but this awaits adequate clinical trials. Other potential approaches would be to combine IFN and BCG or chemotherapeutic agents. The immunomodulator ABPP (2-amino-5-iodo-6-phenyl-4-pyrimidine), which acts as an IFN inducer, has in fact been shown to enhance the activity of BCG against the murine bladder tumor MBT-2 [75]. Preliminary results of a study combining IFN-α and mitomycin C for superficial bladder cancer suggest that the combination may be more effective than either agent alone [76].

## Cervical Cancer and Cervical Intraepithelial Neoplasia

Cervical intraepithelial neoplasia (CIN) is considered to be the forerunner to CIS and invasive cervical carcinoma. It is also known to be associated with human Papillomavirus (HPV) in approximately 90% of cases. IFNs have been demonstrated to induce regression of warts associated with HPV and to effectively treat other Papillomavirus-related diseases such as respiratory papillomatosis [77] suggesting a strong rationale for their use in CIN.

Local treatment of CIN involves destruction of the lesion using cryotherapy and electrocoagulation which is, however, unable to penetrate deep into the tissues treated. IFNs have been injected intralesionally and perilesionally to circumvent this problem, with variable results. Earlier studies [78] reported response rates of up to 100%, but these have been cast in doubt by a recent randomized trial that demonstrated no benefit [79]. Overall, it appears that about half of all patients treated may derive benefit from this form of therapy, many responses being durable. Side effects are generally minimal, in the form of low-grade fevers and myalgias.

Attempts have also been made to use IFNs in combination with other chemotherapeutic agents in the treatment of advanced or recurrent cervical cancers. A recent trial with IFN-α and doxorubicin demonstrated efficacy with tolerable side effects [80].

The effects of IFN-γ and tumor necrosis factor against various cervical carcinoma cell lines have been studied in vitro. In general, growth was inhibited by IFN-γ and to a lesser extent by tumor necrosis factor, with a suggestion of synergy between the two agents [78, 81]. Clinical trials looking at this issue are needed to further define their role in the therapy of cervical cancer.

### Non-Small Cell Lung Cancer (NSCLC)

IFN has been investigated in this disease for three major indications: as therapy for advanced metastatic disease both by itself and as a chemopotentiator, as a radiosensitizer, and as therapy for malignant pleural effusions.

In general, IFN has not been efficacious as systemic therapy for advanced NSCLC. Preclinical data suggested enhancement of the effects of cisplatin on lung cancer xenografts by IFN-α, but a phase II combination of these two agents showed no benefit over cisplatin alone [82]. A study that utilized IFN-β and IFN-γ as pretreatment prior to combination cisplatin and etoposide concluded that efficacy was not enhanced [83]. IFN-α2b when combined with cyclophosphamide, epidoxorubicin and cisplatin produced a 20% response rate and was relatively well tolerated [84]. IFN-β used as a single agent did not result in significant effects in 18 patients with advanced NSCLC.

Work on the effects of IFN-α as radiosensitizer has been done mainly by a group in Helsinki with encouraging results [85], but further study is required. The most impressive effects of IFN have been in the management of recurrent malignant pleural effusion, with clinical and pathological (cytology) improvement reported in a number of studies [86, 87].

### Conclusion

IFNs have been shown to have antitumor clinical activity against a variety of neoplasms over a wide dose range and varied schedules of administration. Overall, IFN-α has been most intensively studied, and has activity that compares favorably with other IFNs. The most encouraging results have been observed in the treatment of melanoma among nonhematologic neoplasms, and applications in locoregional treatment of other tumor types are under active investigation. Of vital importance is the further elucidation of their mechanism of action, to allow a more rational development of this modality in conjunction with other therapies, biologic and chemotherapeutic.

### References


1 Legha SS, Papadopoulos NEJ, Plager C, Ring S, Chawla SP, Evans LM, Benjamin RS: Clinical evaluation of recombinant interferon alfa-2a (Roferon-a) in metastatic melanoma using two different schedules. J Clin Oncol 1987;5:1240–1246.
2 Creagan ET, Ahmann DL, Green SJ, Long HJ, Rubin J, Schutt AJ, Dziewanowski ZE: Phase II study of recombinant leukocyte A interferon (rIFN-αA) in disseminated malignant melanoma. Cancer 1984;54:2844–2849.
3 Robinson WA, Mughal TI, Thomas MR, Johnson M, Spiegel RJ: Treatment of metastatic malignant melonoma with recombinant interferon alpha-2. Immunobiology 1986;172:275–282.
4 Sertoli MR, Bernengo MG, Ardizzoni A, Brunetti I, Falcone A, Vidili MG, Cusimano MP, Appino A, Doveil G, Fortini C, Rosso R: Phase II trial of recombinant alpha-2b interferon in the treatment of metastatic skin melanoma. Oncology 1989;46:96–98.
5 Kirkwood JM, Ernstoff MS: Melanoma: Therapeutic options with recombinant interferons. Semin Oncol 1985;12:7–12.
6 Creagan ET, Ahmann DL, Frytak S, Long HJ, Chang MN, Itri LM: Phase II trials of recombinant leukocyte A interferon in disseminated malignant melanoma: Results in 96 patients. Cancer Treat Rep 1986;70:619–624.
7 Steiner A, Wolf C, Pehamberger H: Comparison of the effects of three different treatment regimens of recombinant interferon (r-IFN alpha, r-IFN gamma, and r-IFN alpha + cimetidine) in disseminated malignant melanoma. J Cancer Res Clin Oncol 1987;113:459–465.
8 von Wussow P, Block B, Hartmann F, Deicher H: Intralesional interferon-alpha therapy in advanced malignant melanoma. Cancer 1988;61:1071–1074.
9 Flodgren P, Borgstrom S, Jonsson PE, Lindstrom C, Sjogren HO: Metastatic malignant melanoma: Regression induced by combined treatment with interferon [HuIFN-alpha(Le)] and cimetidine. Int J Cancer 1983;32:657–665.
10 Creagan ET, Ahmann DL, Green SJ, Long HJ, Frytak S, Itri LM: Phase II study of recombinant leukocyte A interferon (IFN-rA) plus cimetidine in disseminated malignant melanoma. J Clin Oncol 1985;3:977–981.
11 Talpaz M, Plager C, Quesada J, Benjamin R, Kantarjian H, Gutterman J: Difluoromethylornithine and leukocyte interferon: A phase I study in cancer patients. Eur J Cancer Clin Oncol 1986;22:685–689.
12 Croghan MK, Booth A, Meyskens FL Jr: A phase I trial of recombinant interferon-α and α-difluoromethylornithine in metastatic melanoma. J Biol Response Modif 1988;7:409–415.
13 McLeod GRC, Thomson DB, Hersey P: Recombinant interferon alfa-2a in advanced malignant melanoma: A phase I-II study in combination with DTIC. Proc Off Satellite Symp, 14th Int UICC Cancer Congr, Budapest, 1986. Int J Cancer 1987;(suppl 1):31–35.
14 Kirkwood JM, Ernstoff MS, Giuliano A: Clinical trials of interferon alfa-2B (Intron A, alpha-IFN) in melanoma: Review of phase I, II, and III studies. Proc 14th Int Cancer Congr, Budapest Aug 1986.
15 Kirkwood JM, Ernstoff MS, Giuliano A, Gams R, Robinson WA, Costanzi J, Pouillart P, Speyer J, Grimm M, Spiegel R: Interferon alpha 2 and dacarbazine (DTIC) in melanoma. J Natl Cancer Inst 1990;80:1062–1063.

16 Walsh C, Speyer JL, Wernz J, Hochster H, Grossberg H, Chachoua A, Molinaro P, Meyers M, Blum RH: A phase I study of the combination of alpha-2 interferon and cisplatinum. J Biol Response Modif 1989;8:11–15.
17 Wadler S, Einzig AI, Dutcher JP, Ciobanu Landau L, Wiernik PH: Phase II trial of recombinant alpha-2b-interferon and low-dose cyclophosphamide in advanced melanoma and renal cell carcinoma. Am J Clin Oncol 1988;11: 55–59.
18 Miller RL, Steis RG, Clark JW, Smith JW II, Crum E, McKnight JE, Hawkins MJ, Jones MJ, Longo DL, Urba WJ: Randomized trial of recombinant α2b-interferon with or without indomethacin in patients with metastatic malignant melanoma. Cancer Res 1989;49:1871–1876.
19 Ernstoff MS, Trautman T, Davis CA, Reich SD, Witman P, Balser J, Rudnick S, Kirkwood JM: A randomized phase I/II study of continuous versus intermittent intravenous interferon gamma in patients with metastatic melanoma. J Clin Oncol 1987;5;1804–1810.
20 Creagan ET, Ahmann DL, Long HJ, Frytak S, Sherwin SA, Chang MN: Phase II study of recombinant interferon-gamma in patients with disseminated malignant melanoma. Cancer Treat Rep 1987;71:843–844.
21 Osanto S, Jansen R, Naipal AMIH, Gratama JW, van Leeuwen A, Cleton FJ: In vivo effects of combination treatment with recombinant interferon-gamma and -alpha in metastatic melanoma. Int J Cancer 1989;43:1001–1006.
22 Kirkwood JM, Ernstoff MS: Cutaneous melanoma; in DeVita VT Jr, Hellman S, Rosenberg SA (eds): Biologic Therapy of Cancer. Philadelphia, Lippincott, 1991, pp 311–333.
23 Creagan ET, Ahmann DL, Frytak S, Long HJ, Itri LM: Recombinant leukocyte A interferon (rIFN-αA) in the treatment of disseminated malignant melanoma: Analysis of complete and long-term responding patients. Cancer 1986;58:2576–2578.
24 Boring CC, Squires TS, Tong T: Cancer statistics, 1993. CA 1993;43:7–26.
25 DeKernion JB, Lindner A: Treatment of advanced renal cell carcinoma. Prog Clin Biol Res 1982;100:641–659.
26 Muss HB, Welander C, Caponera M, Reavis K, Cruz JM, Cooper R, Jackson DV, Richards F Jr III, Stuart JJ, Spurr CL, White DR, Zekan PJ, Capizzi RL: Interferon and doxorubicin in renal cell carcinoma. Cancer Treat Rep 1985; 69:721–722.
27 Muss HB, Costanzi JJ, Leavitt R, Williams RD, Kempf RA, Pollard R, Ozer H, Zekan PJ, Grunberg SM, Mitchell MS, Caponera M, Gavigan M, Ernst ML, Venturi C, Greiner J, Spiegel RJ: Recombinant alfa interferon in renal cell carcinoma: A randomized trial of two routes of administration. J Clin Oncol 1987;5: 286–291.
28 Belldegrun A, Koo AS, Bochner B, Figlin R, DeKernion JB: Immunotherapy for advanced renal cell cancer: The role of radical nephrectomy. Eur Urol 1990;18 (suppl 2):42–45.
29 Hirsh M, Lipton A, Harvey H, Givant E, Hopper K, Jones G, Zeffren J, Levitt D: Phase I study of interleukin-2 and interferon alfa-2a as outpatient therapy for patients with advanced malignancy. J Clin Oncol 1990;8:1657–1663.
30 Atzpodien J, Korfer A, Franks CR, Poliwada H, Kirchner H: Home therapy with recombinant interleukin-2 and interferon-alpha 2b in advanced human malignancies. Lancet 1990; 335:1509–1512.
31 Ernstoff MS, Nair S, Bahnson RR, Miketic LM, Banner B, Gooding W, Day R, Whiteside T, Hakala T, Kirkwood JM: A phase IA trial of sequential recombinant DNA-produced interferons: Combination recombinant interferon gamma and recombinant interferon alfa in patients with metastatic renal cell carcinoma. J Clin Oncol 1990;8:1637–1649.
32 DeMulder P, Debruyne F, Rikken G, Franssen M, van Hoesel Q, Damsa O: Recombinant (r) tumor necrosis factor alpha (TNF-alpha) and interferon (IFN)-gamma(g) in the treatment of advanced renal cell carcinoma (RCC) (abstract). Proc Am Soc Clin Oncol 1989;8:144.
33 Aapro MS, Alberts DS, Salmon SE: Interactions of human leukocyte interferon with vinca alkaloids and other chemotherapeutic agents against human tumors in clonogenic assay. Cancer Chemother Pharmacol 1983;10:161–168.
34 Fossa SD: Is interferon with or without vinblastine the 'treatment of choice' in metastatic renal cell carcinoma? The Norwegian Radium Hospital's Experience 1983–1986. Semin Surg Oncol 1988;4:178–183.
35 Sertoli MR, Brunetti I, Ardizzoni A, Falcone A, Guarneri D, Boccardo F, Martorana G, Curotto A, Sicignano A, Rosso R, Santi L: Recombinant A-2a interferon plus vinblastine in the treatment of metastatic renal cell carcinoma. Am J Clin Oncol 1989;12:43–45.
36 Gutterman JU, Blumenschein GR, Alexanian R, Yap HY, Buzdar AU, Cabanillas F, Hortobagyi GN, Hersh EM, Rasmussen SL, Harmon M, Kramer M, Pestka S: Leukocyte interferon-induced tumor regression in human metastatic breast cancer, multiple myeloma, and malignant lymphoma. Ann Intern Med 1980;93: 399–405.
37 Sarna GP, Figlin RA: Phase II trial of alpha lymphoblastoid interferon given weekly as a treatment of advanced breast cancer. Cancer Treat Rep 1985;69:547–549.
38 van den Berg HW, Leahey WJ, Lynch M, Clarke R, Nelson J: Recombinant human interferon alpha increases oestrogen receptor expression in human breast cancer cells (ZR-75-1) and sensitizes them to the anti-proliferative effects of tamoxifen. Br J Cancer 1987;55:255–257.
39 Sica G, Iacopino F, Della Cuna GR, Marchetti P: Recombinant interferon-alpha 2b affects proliferation, steroid receptors and sensitivity to tamoxifen of cultured breast cancer cells (CG-5). Anticancer Drugs 1992;3:147–153.
40 Buzzi F, Brugia M, Rossi G, Giustini L, Scoponi C, Sica G: Combination of beta-interferon and tamoxifen as a new way to overcome clinical resistance to tamoxifen in advanced breast cancer. Anticancer Res 1992;12:869–871.
41 Macheledt JE, Buzdar AU, Hortobagyi GN, Frye DK, Gutterman JU, Holmes FA: Phase II evaluation of interferon added to tamoxifen in the treatment of metastatic breast cancer. Breast Cancer Res Treat 1991;18:165–170.
42 Miglietta L, Repetto L, Gardin G, Amoroso D, Giudici S, Naso C, Merlini L, Queirolo P, Campora E, Pronzato P: Tamoxifen and alpha interferon in advanced breast cancer. J Chemother 1991;3:383–386.
43 Buzdar AU, Hortobagyi GN, Kau SWC, Smith TL, Fraschini G, Holmes FA, Gutterman JU, Hug VM, Singletary E, Ames FC, McNeese MD: Adjuvant therapy with escalating doses of doxorubicin and cyclophosphamide with or without leukocyte alfa-interferon for stage II or III breast cancer. J Clin Oncol 1992;10:1540–1546.
44 Ozzello L, Habif DV, DeRosa CM, Cantell K: Cellular events accompanying regression of skin recurrences of breast carcinomas treated with intralesional injections of natural interferons alpha and gamma. Cancer Res 1992;52: 4571–4581.
45 Mazuran R, Ikic-Sutlic M, Jereb B, Stabuc B, Krasovec MU, Cerar O, Soos E: Intraperitoneal application of natural IFN alpha in breast cancer patients with pleural carcinomatosis. Monitoring of immunotherapy by assaying serum interferon levels. J Biol Regul Homeost Agents 1992;6:46–52.
46 Inoue M, Tan YH: Enhancement of actinomycin-D and cis-diamminedichloroplatinum (II)-induced killing of human fibroblasts by human beta-interferon. Cancer Res 1983;43:5484–5487.
47 Giacomini P, Mottolese M, Fraioli R, Benevolo M, Venturo I, Natali PG: Antigenic modulation of metastatic breast and ovarian carcinoma cells by intracavitary injection of IFN-alpha. Br J Cancer 1992;66:342–344.
48 Goldstein D, Laszlo J: Interferon therapy in cancer: From imaginon to interferon. Cancer Res 1986;46:4315–4329.
49 Niloff JM, Knapp RC, Jones G, Schaetzl EM, Bast RC Jr: Recombinant leukocyte alpha interferon in advanced ovarian carcinoma. Cancer Treat Rep 1985;69:895–896.
50 DiSaia PJ, Gillette P: Human lymphoblastoid interferon (IFN alpha-N1) plus doxorubicin, cyclophosphamide, and cisplatin in the treatment of advanced epithelial ovarian malignancies. A phase I-II study of the Gynecologic Oncology Group. Am J Clin Oncol 1991;14: 71–74.
51 Berek JS, Hacker NF, Lichtenstein A, Jung T, Spina C, Knox RM, Brady J, Greene T, Ettinger LM, Lagasse LD, Bonnem EM, Spiegel RJ, Zighelboim J: Intraperitoneal recombinant α-interfeon for 'salvage' immunotherapy in stage III epithelial ovarian cancer: A Gynecologic Oncology Group study. Cancer Res 1985;45: 4447–4453.

52 Nardi M, Cognetti F, Pollera CF, Giulia MD, Lombardi A, Atlante G, Calabresi F: Intraperitoneal recombinant alpha-2-interferon alternating with cisplatin as salvage therapy for minimal residual-disease ovarian cancer: A phase II study. J Clin Oncol 1990;8:1036–1041.
53 Markman M, Berek JS, Blessing JA, McGuire WP, Bell J, Homesley HD: Characteristics of patients with small-volume residual ovarian cancer unresponsive to cisplatin-based ip chemotherapy: Lessons learned from a Gynecologic Oncology Group phase II trial of ip cisplatin and recombinant alpha interferon. Gynecol Oncol 1992;45:3–8.
54 Repetto L, Chiara S, Guido S, Bruzzone M, Oliva C, Ragni N: Intraperitoneal chemotherapy with carboplatin and interferon alpha in the treatment of relapsed ovarian cancer: A pilot study. Anticancer Res 1991;11:1641–1643.
55 Bezwoda WR, Seymour L, Dansey R: Intraperitoneal recombinant interferon-alpha 2b for recurrent malignant ascites due to ovarian cancer. Cancer 1989;64:1029–1033.
56 Bezwoda WR, Golombick T, Dansey R, Keeping J: Treatment of malignant ascites due to recurrent/refractory ovarian cancer: The use of interferon-alpha or interferon-alpha plus chemotherapy in vivo and in vitro. Eur J Cancer 1991;27:1423–1429.
57 Miyoshi T, Ogawa S, Kanamori T, Nobuhara M, Namba M: Interferon potentiates cytotoxic effects of 5-fluorouracil on cell proliferation of established human cell lines originating from neoplastic tissues. Cancer Lett 1983;17:239–247.
58 Elias L, Sandoval JM: Interferon effects upon fluorouracil metabolism by HL-60 cells. Biochem Biophys Res Commun 1989;163:867–874.
59 Lindley C, Bernard S, Gavigan M, Kaluzny B, Meadows L: Interferon-alpha increases 5-fluorouracil (5-FU) plasma levels 64-fold within one hour: Results of a phase I study (abstract). J Interferon Res 1990;10:II6–31.
60 Wadler S, Schwartz El, Goldman M, Lyver A, Rader M, Zimmerman M, Itri L, Weinberg V, Wiernik PH: Fluorouracil and recombinant alfa-2a-interferon: An active regimen against advanced colorectal carcinoma. J Clin Oncol 1989;7:1769–1775.
61 Wadler S, Wiernik PH: Clinical update on the role of fluorouracil and recombinant interferon alfa-2a in the treatment of colorectal carcinoma. Semin Oncol 1990;17(suppl 1):16–21.
62 Pazdur R, Ajani JA, Patt YZ, Winn R, Jackson D, Shepard B, DeBrow R, Campos L, Quaraishi M, Faintuch J, Abbruzzese JL, Gutterman J, Levin B: Phase II study of fluorouracil and recombinant interferon alfa-2a in previously untreated advanced colorectal carcinoma. J Clin Oncol 1990;8:2027–2031.
63 Preiss J: Fluorouracil plus interferon + folinic acid in regional and systemic therapy in colorectal cancer. Semin Oncol 1992;19(suppl 3): 220–224.
64 Schmoll HJ, Kohne-Wompner CH, Hiddemann W, Knipp H, Wilke H, Bodenstein H, Schoffski P, Bokemeyer C, Lohrmann HP, Preiss J, Kaufer C, Fischer JT, Balleisen L, Urbanitz D, Harstrick A, Hill H: Interferon alpha-2b, 5-fluorouracil, and folinic acid combination therapy in advanced colorectal cancer: Preliminary results of a phase I/II trial. Semin Oncol 1992;19(suppl 3):191–196.
65 Lamm DL: Diagnosis and treatment of bladder cancer. Anticancer Drugs 1992;3(suppl 1):39–47.
66 Glashan RW: A randomized controlled study of intravesical alpha-2b-interferon in carcinoma in situ of the bladder. J Urol 1990;144:658–661.
67 Frangos DN, Killion JJ, Fan D, Fishbeck R, von Eschenbach AC, Fidler IJ: The development of liposomes containing interferon alpha for the intravesical therapy of human superficial bladder cancer. J Urol 1990;143:1252–1256.
68 Hoeltl W, Hasun R, Albrecht W: Prospective randomized trial to evaluate high- versus low-dose interferon-alpha 2b versus conventional chemotherapy in prevention of the recurrence of superficial transitional cell carcinoma of the urinary bladder. Anticancer Drugs 1992;3 (suppl 1):29–32.
69 Seretta V, Pavone C, Corselli G, Pavone-Macaluso: A pilot study comparing different dose levels and administration schedules of interferon-alpha 2b combined with epirubicin for the prevention of recurrence in bladder cancer. Anticancer Drugs 1992;3 (suppl 1):19–23.
70 Sarosdy M: High-dose versus low-dose intravesical interferon-alpha 2b in the treatment of carcinoma in situ: A randomized, controlled study. Anticancer Drugs 1992;3 (suppl 1):13–17.
71 Ferrari P, Castagnetti G, Pollastri CA, Ferrari G, Tavoni F, Grassi D: Chemoimmunotherapy for prophylaxis of recurrence in superficial bladder cancer: Interferon-alpha 2b versus interferon-alpha 2b with epirubicin. Anticancer Drugs 1992;3 (suppl 1):25–27.
72 Logothetis CJ, Hossan E, Sella A, Dexeus FH, Amato RJ: Fluorouracil and recombinant human interferon alfa-2a in the treatment of metastatic chemotherapy-refractory urothelial tumors. J Natl Cancer Inst 1991;83:285–288.
73 Hawkyard SJ, Jackson AM, James K, Prescott S, Smyth JF, Chisholm GD: The inhibitory effects of interferon gamma on the growth of bladder cancer cells. J Urol 1992;147:1399–1403.
74 Hawkyard S, James K, Prescott S, Jackson AM, Ritchie AW, Smyth JF: The effects of recombinant human interferon-gamma on a panel of human bladder cancer cell lines. J Urol 1991; 145:1078–1081.
75 Sarosdy MF, Kierum CA: Combination immunotherapy of murine transitional cell cancer using BCG and an interferon-inducing pyrimidinone. J Urol 1989;142:1376–1379.
76 Engelmann U, Knopf HJ, Graff J: Interferon-alpha 2b instillation prophylaxis in superficial bladder cancer – a prospective, controlled three-armed trial. Project Group Bochum – interferon and superficial bladder cancer. Anticancer Drugs 1992;3 (suppl 1):33–37.
77 Weck PK, Brandsma JL, Whisnant JK: Interferons in the treatment of human papillomavirus diseases. Cancer Metastasis Rev 1986;5: 139–165.
78 Scorticatti CH, de la Pena NC, Bellora OG, Mariotto RA, Casabe AR, Comolli R: Systemic IFN-alpha treatment of multiple bladder papilloma grade I or II patients: Pilot study. J Interferon Res 1982;2:339 343.
79 Frost L, Skajaa K, Hvidmann LE, Fay SJ, Larsen PM: No effect of intralesional injection of interferon on moderate cervical intraepithelial neoplasia. Br J Obstet Gynaecol 1990;97:626–630.
80 Welander CE, Homesley HD, Barrett RJ: Combined interferon alfa and doxorubicin in the treatment of advanced cervical cancer. Am J Obstet Gynecol 1991;165:284–290.
81 Mutch DG, Massed LS, Kao MS, Collins JL: Proliferative and antiproliferative effects of interferon-gamma and tumor necrosis factor-alpha on cell lines derived from cervical and ovarian malignancies. Am J Obstet Gynecol 1990;163:1920–1924.
82 Rosell R, Carles J, Ariza A, Moreno I, Ribelles N, Solano V, Pellicer I, Barnadas A, Abad A: A phase II study of days 1 and 8 cisplatin and recombinant alpha-2b interferon in advanced non-small cell lung cancer. Cancer 1991;67: 2448–2453.
83 Schiller JH, Storer B, Dreicer R, Rosenquist D, Frontiera M, Carbone PP: Randomized phase II-III trial of combination beta and gamma interferons and etoposide and cisplatin in operable non-small cell cancer of the lung. J Natl Cancer Inst 1989;81:1739–1743.
84 Ardizzoni A, Rosso R, Salvati F, Scagliotti G, Soresi E, Ferrara G, Pennucci C, Baldini E, Cruciani AR, Antilli A: Combination chemotherapy and interferon alpha 2b in the treatment of advanced non-small cell lung cancer. The Italian Lung Cancer Task Force (FONICAP). Am J Clin Oncol 1991;14:120–123.
85 Maasilta P, Holsti LR, Halme M, Kivisaari L, Cantell K, Mattson K: Natural alpha-interferon in combination with hyperfractionated radiotherapy in the treatment of non-small cell lung cancer. Int J Radiat Oncol Biol Phys 1992; 23:863–868.
86 Tercelj-Zorman M, Mermolja M, Jereb M, Oman M, Soos E, Petric-Grabnar G, Jereb B: Human leukocyte interferon alpha (HLI-alpha) for treatment of pleural effusion caused by non-small cell lung cancer. A pilot study. Acta Oncol 1991;30:963–965.
87 Rosso R, Rimoldi R, Salvati F, DePalma M, Cinquegrana A, Nicolo G, Ardizzoni A, Fusco U, Capaccio A, Centofanti R: Intrapleural natural beta interferon in the treatment of malignant pleural effusion. Oncology 1988;45:253–256.

Oncology 1994;51:137–141

*Akio Urabe*

Division of Hematology,
Kanto Teishin Hospital, Tokyo, Japan

# Interferons for the Treatment of Hematological Malignancies

**Key Words**
Interferon
Multiple myeloma
Chronic myelogenous leukemia
Hairy cell leukemia
Adult T cell leukemia

**Abstract**
Interferon (IFN) has diverse acitvities against the proliferation and function of various tumor cells. Recently, IFN-α has been widely used in the treatment of several hematological malignancies including chronic myelogenous leukemia (CML), multiple myeloma, and hairy cell leukemia. IFN-α is becoming a first-choice drug in the treatment of CML, because it has been reported to suppress or abolish the $Ph^1$ chromosome in CML patients. IFN-α is used in combination with conventional chemotherapeutic regimens in the treatment of multiple myeloma. There are many ongoing trials that include IFN-α in their regimens to determine whether or not the prognosis of multiple myeloma can be improved. Although the precise mechanism of the action of IFN has not been fully explained, the clinical applications of IFN for various hematological malignancies are expanding.

## Introduction

Interferon (IFN) has been found to inhibit the proliferation of viruses [1]. IFNs now include a class of glycoproteins produced by various cells in response to viral infections, specific antigens or mitogens. There are three major IFNs: α, β, and γ. IFN-α is predominantly produced by virus-stimulated leukocytes. IFN-β mainly by fibroblasts, and IFN-γ by T lymphocytes. IFNs have not only antiviral activity but also antineoplastic activity, although the precise mechanisms of action are obscure. The in vitro growth of embryonic tissue, the lymphoid system and fibroblasts is inhibited in the presence of IFNs. The cell growth of some hematological malignancies is also inhibited by the addition of IFNs, and recently, IFNs have been used in their treatment. This article reviews the clinical usefulness of IFNs for hematological malignancies.

## Multiple Myeloma

IFN-α has been used in the treatment of multiple myeloma since 1979. At first, it was used alone to induce remission or as salvage therapy, but its efficacy was minimal. Recently, combination therapy using IFN-α and cytotoxic drugs, and maintenance therapy with IFNα have been tried, and hopeful results have been reported.

### *In vitro Effects of IFN*

When myeloma cells were incubated with IFN, their viability was generally suppressed, although this result was not obtained in all cases [2]. However, the immunoglobulin level in the culture medium was always decreased, and it was speculated that the decrease in immunoglobulin production in response to IFN was not always related to the cytotoxic effect [2]. The incorporation of $^3$H-TdR into myeloma cells was not always suppressed by the addition of IFN, but the production of M protein decreased in proportion to the amount of IFN added [3].

Akio Urabe, MD
Division of Hematology, Kanto Teishin Hospital
5-9-22 Higashi-Gotanda
Shinagawa-ku
Tokyo 141 (Japan)


0030–2414/94/0512–0137
$5.00/0

*Induction of Remission by Treatment with IFN Alone*

There are many reports of treatment with IFN alone to induce remission in fresh cases of multiple myeloma [4–7]. The efficacy rate of IFN alone was around 15%, which is not as good as MP (melphalan plus prednisone) or VMCP (vincristine, melphalan, cyclophosphamide and prednisone). It was speculated from these studies that IgA- or IgD-type myeloma and patients with a relatively small tumor burden responded well.

*Salvage Therapy with IFN Alone*

There are several reports of salvage therapy with IFN alone in refractory or relapsed cases of multiple myeloma [8–10]. Efficacy rates were between 11 and 26%, and improvement of bone pain or physical activity was obtained even though patients did not reach the criteria of effectiveness.

*Maintenance Therapy*

There has been controversy as to whether or not maintenance therapy is necessary in patients with multiple myeloma in remission. Mandelli et al. [11] have reported that maintenance with IFN-α ($3 \times 10^6$ U/m$^2$ three times a week) prolonged remission and survival when compared with no maintenance therapy [11]. It is possible that maintenance therapy with IFN-α might improve the prognosis of myeloma patients.

*Combination Therapy with Conventional Chemotherapy and IFN*

IFN-α in combination with prednisone or cyclophosphamide suppresses the colony formation of myeloma cells in vitro additively, and IFN-α in combination with melphalan acts synergistically [9]. Moreover, the combination of IFN-α, melphalan and prednisone can suppress colony formation at low concentrations of each drug.

Based upon such experimental data, the clinical application of IFN-α in combination with conventional chemotherapy has been tried in many institutions. However, most of the trials were carried out on refractory cases, and the efficacy was not as good as expected. Therefore, trials using combination therapy with IFN-α and cytotoxic drugs were extended to fresh cases of multiple myeloma. Cooper et al. [12] reported that a combination of IFN-α, melphalan and prednisone resulted in remission in 75% (18/24) of fresh cases of myeloma. Montuoro et al. [13] compared the efficacy of MP with MP plus IFN in fresh cases, and reported that the remission rate was 68% in the MP group and 95% in the MP-IFN group. Recently, Mellstedt et al. [14] reported that the efficacy rate of MP plus IFN-α in stage II myeloma was 76% compared with 48% for MP alone. Moreover, the efficacy of MP plus IFN-α was extremely good: 91% in IgA myeloma compared with 52% for MP alone. On the other hand, there was no difference in efficacy between MP and MP plus IFN-α in IgG or Bence Jones protein types.

Many studies of multiple myeloma have tried to introduce IFN-α in combination with various conventional chemotherapeutic regimens to induce remission or as maintenance chemotherapy. Most of the results suggest that IFN-α acts synergistically in combination with cytotoxic drugs, and convincing data are now accumulating.

## Chronic Myelogenous Leukemia

The most fundamental drugs in the treatment of chronic myelogenous leukemia (CML) have long been busulfan and hydroxyurea. These drugs can reduce the white blood cell count and splenomegaly, but cannot alter disease progression to blastic crisis. Bone marrow transplantation is the only therapy for CML that can bring about cure. However, it is not always available for all patients.

Recently, IFN has been introduced in the treatment of CML, and it has been suggested that IFN may eliminate or reduce the Ph$^1$ chromosome in CML patients.

*Ph$^1$ Chromosome and CML*

The Ph$^1$ chromosome is observed in more than 95% of CML patients. It results from a translocation between chromosome 9 and chromosome 22, that is t(9;22)(q34;q11). A new fusion gene called bcr-abl is formed on the break point of the shortened arm of 22q. The bcr-abl gene produces a specific protein which should be fundamentally related with the pathogenesis of CML.

*IFN Therapy of CML*

Since Talpaz et al. [15] reported the results that the administration of IFN-α reduced or eliminated the Ph$^1$ chromosome in CML patients, it has become a hopeful drug in the treatment of CML. The efficacy of IFN-α was examined using hematological and cytogenetic criteria [16]. The administration of IFN-α alone resulted in hematological remission in 77.9% (70/96) of patients with CML, and complete disappearance of the Ph$^1$ chromosome was confirmed in at least one examination in 18.8% (18/96) of the patients [17]. Preliminary data on the relationship between the cytogenetic effect and disease-free survival have been reported [17]. IFN-α administration

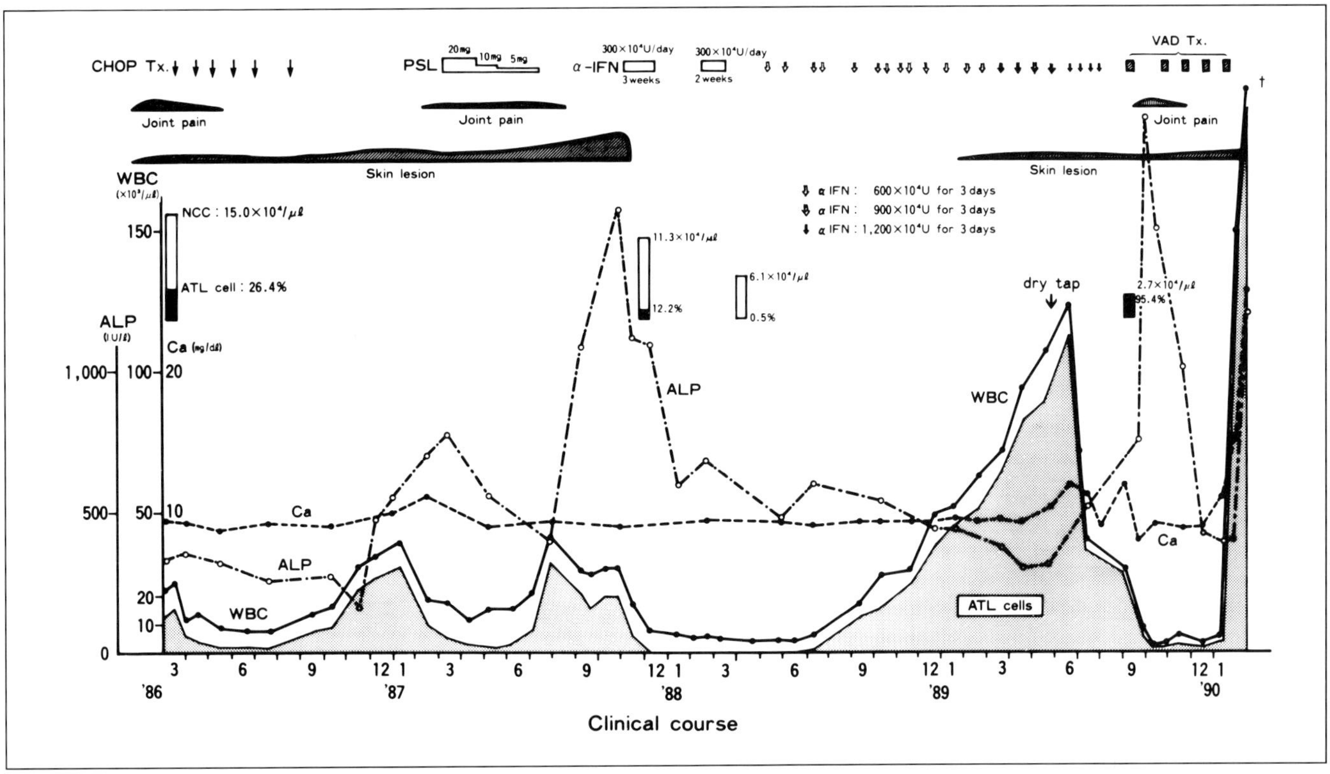

1

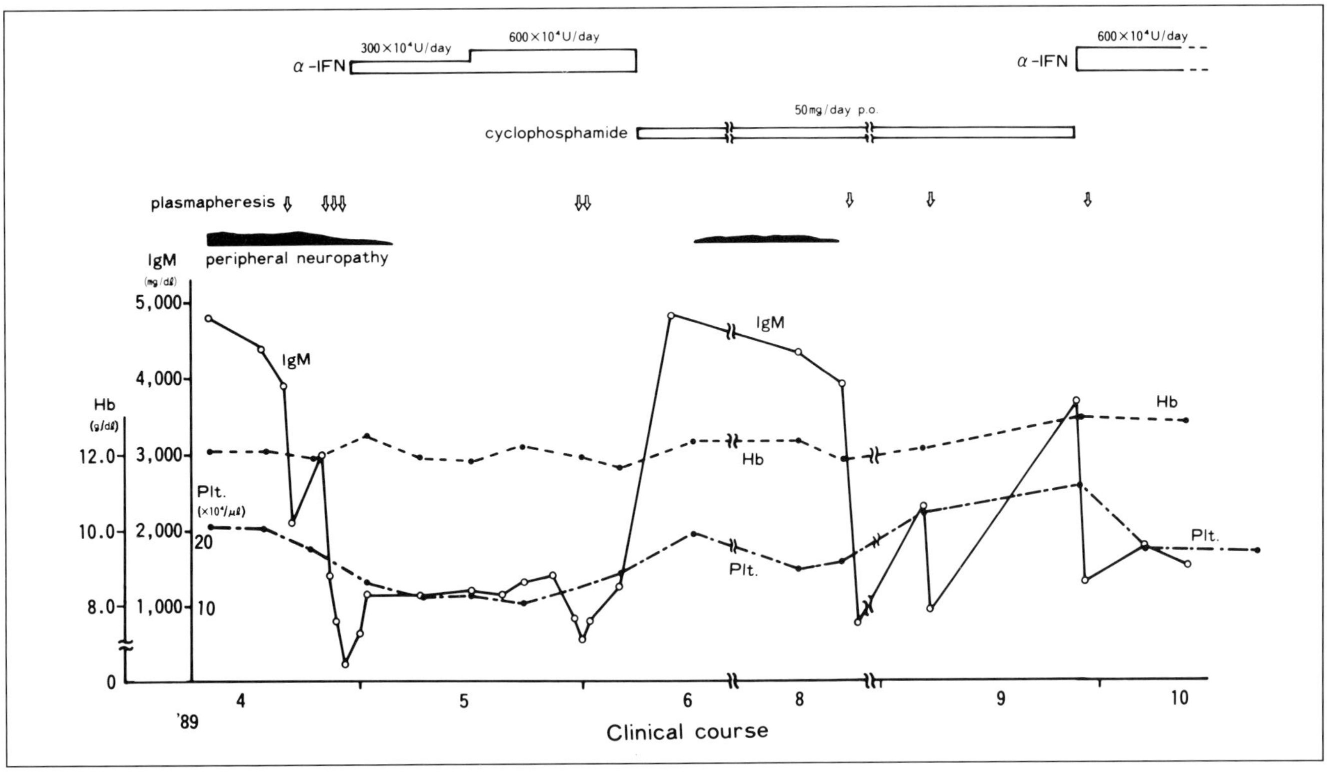

2

**Fig. 1.** Clinical course of a 39-year-old female with adult T cell leukemia (ATL). The growth of ATL cells was suppressed by the administration of IFN-α.

**Fig. 2.** Clinical course of a 63-year-old male with macroglobulinemia. IgM production was suppressed by the administration of IFN-α.

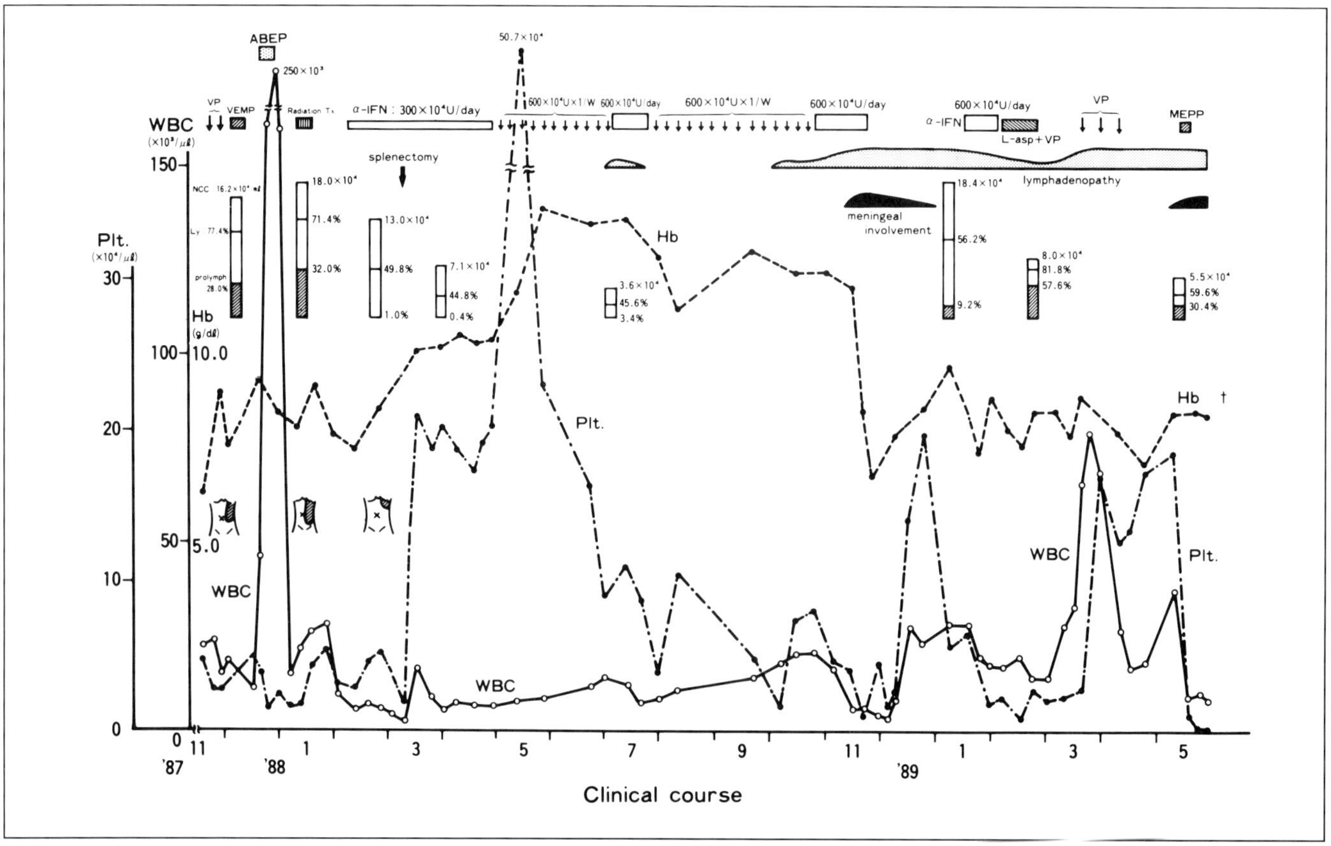


**Fig. 3.** Clinical course of a 44-year-old male with chronic lymphocytic leukemia in prolymphocytoid transformation. Splenomegaly and leukocytosis were suppressed by the administration of IFN-α.

has also been tried in relapsed cases after bone marrow transplantation, and hematological or cytogenetic remission was confirmed in some of the cases [18, 19]. Higano et al. [19] treated 18 patients with CML who had relapsed after allogeneic bone marrow transplantation with IFN-α ($3 \times 10^6 - 6 \times 10^6$ U/m$^2$) every day, and have reported that in 6 patients (33%) the Ph[1] chromosome had completely disappeared, and 2 had a partial response. It was reported that IFN-α was also effective in the accelerated phase of CML, and suppression of the Ph[1] chromosome was also observed [20]. Additional chromosome abnormalities were eliminated by increasing the dose of IFN-α [21].

The precise mechanism of the effectiveness of IFN-α in therapy for CML is obscure. The mechanism involved in suppressing the Ph[1] chromosome is also unknown. IFN-α can suppress in vitro colony formation of CFU-Meg, CFU-GM and BFU-E. One report speculated that the clinical efficacy of IFN-α was related to its suppression of colony formation in vitro [22].

IFN-γ also has clinical efficacy in CML, but there are fewer reported cases using IFN-γ. Because IFN-α and IFN-γ have different receptors, they may achieve their effects via different mechanisms.

There are many unresolved problems in the IFN treatment of CML. Is it important to use IFN in inducing remission or in maintenance therapy? The appropriate dose of IFN in maintenance therapy is also unknown. The most important thing to determine must be how the prognosis of patients with CML is improved by the administration of IFN.

## Other Hematological Malignancies

IFN has been used in hematological malignancies other than myeloma and CML: hairy cell leukemia, adult T cell leukemia, chronic lymphocytic leukemia, macroglobulinemia, and essential thrombocythemia.

IFN-α is now considered a standard choice of therapy for hairy cell leukemia [23]. There are many studies reporting the efficacy of IFN-α2a and IFN-α2b in the treatment of hairy cell leukemia. When the results of several independent groups of investigators were combined, the overall response rate was 89%, of which 9% were complete, 71% partial, and 10% minor [24]. Initial complete responses were rare but partial responses were common in many studies. Although IFN-α does not produce curative complete remission in hairy cell leukemia as a single agent, it is effective and highly active in its treatment. Twelve months of IFN-α therapy at a dose of $2 \times 10^6$ U/$m^2$ subcutaneously three times a week is recommended. Hairy cell leukemia patients who underwent splenectomy after achievement of complete remission after IFN-α therapy have also been reported [25].

IFN-α is effective in adult T cell leukemia patients, especially those who have skin eruptions [26]. IFN-α is also effective in essential thrombocythemia, macroglobulinemia and some cases of chronic lymphocytic leukemia. Clinical courses of typical cases are shown in figures 1–3.

## References


1 Isaacs A, Lindenmann J: Virus interference. I. The interferon. Proc R Soc B (Lond) 1957;147:258–267.
2 Grandér D, von Stedingk LV, von Stedingk M, Wasserman J, Einhorn S: Influence of interferon on antibody production and viability of malignant cells from patients with multiple myeloma. Eur J Haematol 1991;46:17–25.
3 Tanaka H, Tanabe O, Iwato K, Asaoku H, Ishikawa H, Nobuyoshi M, Kawano M, Kuramoto A: Sensitive inhibitory effect of interferon-alfa on M-protein secretion of human myeloma cells. Blood 1989;74:1718–1722.
4 Mellstedt H, Ahre A, Björkholm M, Holm G, Johansson B, Strander H: Interferon therapy in myelomatosis. Lancet 1979;i:245–247.
5 Ahre A, Björkholm M, Mellstedt H, Brenning G, Engstedt L, Gahrton G, Gyllenhammar H, Holm G, Johansson B, Järnmark M, Karnström L, Killander A, Lerner R, Lockner D, Lönnqvist B, Nilsson B, Simonsson B, Stalfelt AM, Strander H, Svedmyr E, Wadman B, Wedelin C: Human leukocyte interferon and intermittent high-dose melphalan-prednisone administration in the treatment of multiple myeloma: A randomized clinical trial from the myeloma group of central Sweden. Cancer Treat Rep 1984;68:1331–1338.
6 Ludwig H, Cortelezzi A, Scheithauer W, Van Camp BGK, Kuzmits R, Fillet G, Peetermans M, Polli E, Flener R: Recombinant interferon alfa-2C versus polychemotherapy (VMCP) for treatment of multiple myeloma: A prospective randomized trial. Eur J Cancer Clin Oncol 1986;22:1111–1116.
7 Quesada JR, Alexanian R, Hawkins M, Barlogie B, Borden E, Itri L, Gutterman U: Treatment of multiple myeloma with recombinant α-interferon. Blood 1986;67:275–278.
8 Costanzi JJ, Cooper MR, Scarffe JH, Ozer H, Grubbs SS, Ferraresi RW, Pollard RB, Spiegel J: Phase II study of recombinant alpha-2 interferon in resistant multiple myeloma. J Clin Oncol 1985;3:654–659.
9 Cooper MR, Welander CE: Interferons in the treatment of multiple myeloma. Cancer 1987; 59:594–600.
10 Ohno R: Interferons in the treatment of multiple myeloma. Int J Cancer 1987;(suppl 1):14–20.
11 Mandelli F, Avvisati G, Amadori S, Boccadoro M, Gernone A, Lauta VM, Marmont F, Petrucci MT, Tirbalto M, Vegna ML, Dammacco F, Pileri A: Maintenance treatment with recombinant interferon alfa-2b in patients with multiple myeloma responding to conventional induction chemotherapy. N Engl J Med 1990; 322:1430–1434.
12 Cooper MR, Fefer A, Thompson J, Case DC Jr, Kempf R, Sacher R, Neefe J, Bickers J, Scarffe JH, Spiegel R, Bonnem E: Alpha-2-interferon/melphalan/prednisone in previously untreated patients with multiple myeloma: A phase I–II trial. Cancer Treat Rep 1986;70:473–376.
13 Montuoro A, De Rosa L, De Blasio A, Picilli L, Petti N, De Laurenzi A: Alpha-2a interferon/melphalan/prednisone versus melphalan/prednisone in previously untreated patients with multiple myeloma. Br J Haematol 1990;76: 365–368.
14 Mellstedt H, Österborg, A, Björkholm M, Björeman M, Brenning G, Gahrton G, Grimfors G, Gyllenhammar H, Hast R, Juliusson G, Järnmark M, Killander A, Kimby E, Lerner R, Merk K, Ohrling M, Simonsson B, Smedmyr B, Stalfelt AM, Strander H, Svedmyr E, Uden AM, Wadman D, Osby E: Treatment of multiple myeloma with interferon alpha: The Scandinavian experience. Br J Haematol 1991; 79(suppl 1):21–25.
15 Talpaz M, McCredie KB, Mavligit GM, Gutterman JU: Leukocyte interferon-induced myeloid cytoreduction in chronic myelogenous leukemia. Blood 1983;62:689–692.
16 Talpaz M, Kantarjian HM, McCredie KB, Keating MJ, Trujillo J, Gutterman J: Clinical investigation of human alpha interferon in chronic myelogenous leukemia. Blood 1987; 69:1280–1288.
17 Talpaz M, Kantarjian H, Kurzrock R, Trujillo JM, Gutterman JU: Interferon-alpha produces sustained cytogenetic responses in chronic myelogenous leukemia. Ann Intern Med 1991; 114:532–538.
18 Arcese W, Mauro FR, Screnci M, Alimena G, Iori AP, De Cuia MR, Lo Coco F, Montefusco E, Fazi P, Mandelli F: Alpha-2b-interferon as single therapy for patients with chronic myeloid leukemia relapsing after T-cell depleted allogeneic bone marrow transplantation. Eur J Haematol 1990;45(suppl 52):36–39.
19 Higano CS, Raskind WH, Singer JW: Use of α interferon for the treatment of relapse of chronic myelogenous leukemia in chronic phase after allogeneic bone marrow transplantation. Blood 1992;80:1437–1442.
20 Ogura H, Tani K, Kozai Y, Watari K, Kodo H, Ozawa K, Asano S, Takaku F: Effect of interferon-α in patients with chronic myelogenous leukemia in the accelerated phase: Cytogenetic and molecular studies. Jpn J Cancer Res 1990; 81:682–686.
21 Claxton D, Kantarjian H, Kurzrock R, Trujillo JM, Gutterman JU, Talpaz M: Alpha interferon dose-dependent suppression of secondary clones in a patient with Philadelphia-positive chronic myelogenous leukemia. Acta Haematol 1990;83:149–151.
22 Geissler D, Gastl G, Aulitzky W, Tilg H, Gaggl S, Konwalinka G, Huber C: Recombinant interferon-alpha-2C in chronic myelogenous leukemia: Relationship of sensitivity of committed haematopoietic precursor cell in vitro (BFU-E, CFU-GM, CFU-Meg) and clinical response. Leuk Res 1990;14:629–636.
23 Quesada JR, Gutterman JU, Hersh EM: Treatment of hairy cell leukemia with alpha interferons. Cancer 1986;57:1678–1680.
24 Saven A, Piro LD: Treatment of hairy cell leukemia. Blood 1992;79:1111–1120.
25 Pangalis GA, Boussiotis VA, Kittas C, Panayiotidis PA, Loukopoulos D, Fessas P: Hairy cell leukemia: Splenectomy after alpha 2b-interferon therapy. Blood 1991;78:1385.
26 Ohbayashi Y, Urabe A, Niitani K: Adult T-cell leukemia and interferon alpha. Ann Intern Med 1988;109:992.

Oncology 1994;51:142–153

*Udo Hieber*[a]
*Manfred E. Heim*[b]

[a] III. Medizinische Klinik, Onkologisches Zentrum, Klinikum Mannheim, and
[b] Sonnenberg-Klinik, Bad Sooden-Allendorf, BRD

# Tumor Necrosis Factor for the Treatment of Malignancies

**Key Words**
Tumor necrosis factor
Cytokine, combination therapy
Anticancer agents
Neoplasms, therapy

**Abstract**
Tumor necrosis factor (TNF) is a cytokine produced in vivo by activated macrophages and monocytes with pleiotropic effects on normal and malignant cells. TNF is cytotoxic to several tumor cell lines in vitro and in vivo. Phase I and phase II trials have been conducted to determine toxicity to humans and to evaluate responses. Recent investigations will be reviewed. Despite promising results in vitro and in vivo, data from systemic administration in the treatment of malignancies have been disappointing. Local administration has been successful. Therefore, we suggest that future efforts concerning TNF administration in the treatment of malignancies should aim at local treatment.

## Introduction

Tumor necrosis factor (TNF) is a typical cytokine, secreted by cells of the monocyte/macrophage lineage (monokine), with antineoplastic activity. It possesses a wide range of cell regulatory, immune and inflammatory properties that overlap with other members of the cytokine network such as interleukin-1 (IL-1) and interferon-γ (IFN-γ) [1]. The phenomenon that certain cancer patients who developed concurrent bacterial infections would also experience remissions of their malignant disease was already recognized in the late 1700s. A case history of a patient who had a regression of a recurrent lymphosarcoma under the influence of an erysipelas led Coley, a New York surgeon, to treat his patients with malignant diseases with a filtered medium of bacterial cultures of *Streptococcus pyogenes* and *Serratia marcescens.* [2]. Until the 1930s Coley's toxins were the only recognized therapeutic agents in cancer therapy before being replaced by the more quantifiable techniques of chemotherapy and radiotherapy. Fifty years later it was demonstrated that *S. marcescens* extracts induced characteristic hemorrhage and necrosis in transplanted sarcomas in mice [3]. The active component of the extract was purified and identified as a lipopolysaccharide (LPS) from the bacteria cell wall. Carswell et al. [4] reported the existence of a 'tumor necrosis factor' in the serum of Bacillus Calmette-Guérin (BCG)-treated mice, which induced hemorrhagic necrosis in subcutaneous Meth A sarcoma transplanted tumors. There was some evidence that the cells responsible for TNF in vivo were macrophages which in the activated state were highly responsive to LPS stimulation. With an appropriate stimulation of activated macrophages or monocytic cell lines it was possible to synthesize TNF and to release it into the culture medium. TNF production was also observed in other animals and in humans [5, 6].

Dr. U. Hieber
III. Medizinische Klinik
Onkologisches Zentrum, Klinikum Mannheim
Postfach 10 00 23
D–68305 Mannheim (FRG)


0030–2414/94/0512–0142
$5.00/0

This serum was directly cytotoxic for some tumor cell lines in vitro, including the L929 mouse fibrosarcoma line, and this helped to provide a rapid assay for TNF activity in vitro. Protein purification and partial sequencing led to the cloning of human TNF and purified protein production by recombinant DNA technology followed in 1985 [7].

In the early 1980s Beutler et al. [8] identified a protein they called 'cachectin' which was associated with chronic wasting disorders and sepsis. In 1985, cachectin was purified and isolated. Based on sequence analysis, it became clear that TNF and cachectin were the same molecule [9]. Lymphotoxin (LT), a tumorlytic protein produced by lymphocytes, was also purified, identified and cloned in the early 1980s [19]. It is 32% homologous with TNF, appears to act at the same receptor and was called TNF-β. Generally it shows activities identical to TNF-α, except in a few cases where it is less or not active. Both the TNF and the LT gene are located on human chromosome 6 near the HLA locus [11].

TNF receptors are present on nearly all cell types with a few exceptions, such as erythrocytes and unstimulated T lymphocytes. A correlation between the number of receptors and the magnitude of response has not be seen. Recently two types of TNF receptor have been recognized [12–14]. One has a molecular weight of about 55 kD (TNF-R55 or TNF-RI), the other has a molecular weight of about 75 kD (TNF-R75 or TNF-RII). While TNF-RI seems to be ubiquitous, TNF-RII seems to appear more on cells of hematopoietic origin. [15–17]. The number of TNF receptors per cell is actively regulated. Type I interferons and IFN-γ increase the expression of cell surface receptors. This increase does not cause an alteration in binding affinity or changes in sensitivity in TNF cytolysis [18]. The number of TNF receptors is down-regulated by IL-1, LPS, phorbol esters and other activators of protein kinase C [19–22]. These alterations are associated with decreased TNF sensitivity.

The exact mechanism of the antitumor action of TNF is unknown. There are direct antitumoral effects in vitro observed for TNF alone. The cytotoxicity of TNF is potentiated by other agents (cytokines, chemotherapeutics, radiation and hyperthermia). Effects on endothelial cells and induction of procoagulation can lead to acute hemorrhagic necrosis in tumor models. TNF is an activator and a mediator of macrophage and natural killer (NK) cell tumoricidal action. In some systems, TNF can induce tumor-specific immunity [23]. There appear to be multiple mechanisms for cellular resistance to the antiproliferative effects of TNF. Cells pretreated with cytokines are 10- to 100-fold less sensitive to the effects of TNF-α or TNF-β. The presence of gap junctions has been associated with resistance; a cross-resistance has been reported with doxorubicin in human breast carcinoma. Cells with amplified expression of the oncogene HER2/ERB-B2 also seem to be associated with resistance [23].

**Table 1.** Agents shown to be synergistically cytotoxic with TNF in vitro

| |
|---|
| Interferon-α, -β, and -γ |
| Interleukin-4 |
| Hyperthermia |
| Inhibitors of mRNA synthesis |
| Actinomycin D |
| 5-Fluorouracil |
| Mitosis inhibitors |
| Alkylating agents |
| Cyclophosphamide |
| Cisplatin |
| Ionizing radiation |
| Topoisomerase II inhibitors |
| Doxorubicin |
| Mitoxantrone |
| Etoposide |
| Amsacrine |

Modified from Spriggs [23].

## Preclinical Effects of TNF

TNF has an antiproliferative effect against several transformed neoplastic cell lines in vitro. These are generally measured by growth inhibition or cytotoxic assays. The most common assay utilizes L929 mouse transformed fibroblasts. A variety of tumor cell lines is found to be sensitive to TNF, e.g., astrocytoma, breast cancer, colon carcinoma, cervical carcinoma, ovarian cancer, lung cancer, and melanoma. Some other tumor cell lines showed no response to TNF. Among these are bladder tumors, several lung tumors and melanoma cell lines, sarcomas, one cervical and one colon cancer cell line [23]. Most non-small cell and small cell lung cancers are also resistant to TNF combined with topoisomerase-II-targeted drugs (etoposide and doxorubicin) [24]. A list of TNF drug synergies is shown in table 1. In investigations of the last 3 years, antiproliferative effects have been reported on several more tumor cell lines, summarized in table 2. Several hematological malignancies are known to

**Table 2.** Investigations with TNF in human and non-human cell lines

| Author | Cell line | Growth inhibition by TNF[1] | Combination | Augmentation of cytotoxic effect[1] | Remarks |
|---|---|---|---|---|---|
| *TNF* | | | | | |
| Iwasaka et al. [27] | human cervical adenocarcinoma | 1/5 | none | | |
| van de Loosdrecht et al. [28] | human histiocytic lymphoma | 1/1 | none | | |
| Sherwood et al. [29] | human prostatic cancer | 3/3 | none | | |
| *TNF in combination with other cytokines* | | | | | |
| Hand et al. [30] | human mesothelioma | 0/3 | IFN-γ | 3/3 | 2/3 cell lines were mildly sensitive to IFN-γ alone |
| Bowman et al. [31] | human mesothelioma | 0/5 | IFN-α | 1/5 | minor growth inhibition with IFN-α (5/5) |
| Denis and Ghadirian [32] | murine mastocytoma | 0/1 | IFN-γ | 1/1 | combinations with GM-CSF, and IFN-α: no augmentation |
| Eisenthal and McIntosh [33] | melanoma | 0/1 | IL-2 | 1/1 | addition of B16 melanoma antibodies increased anti-tumor effect |
| Raitano et al. [34] | human pancreas carcinoma | 1/5 | IFN-γ | 2/5 | |
| Sacchi et al. [35] | squamous cell carcinoma, head and neck | 3/12 | IFN-α<br>IFN-γ | 10/12<br>6/7 | |
| Massad et al. [36] | human cervical carcinoma<br>human ovarian carcinoma | 0/5<br>0/3 | | 4/5<br>3/3 | augmented effect in presence of protein synthesis inhibitors |
| Hoon et al. [37] | human renal carcinoma | 0/5 | IL-4 | 5/5 | |
| *TNF in combination with cytotoxic agents* | | | | | |
| Bonavida et al. [38] | human ovarian carcinoma | 0/4 | adriamycin | 1/4 | one adriamycin-resistant cell line responded |
| Vigani et al. [39] | human ovarian carcinoma | 1/1 | mitoxantrone | 1/1 | |
| Schiller and Bittner [40] | human colon carcinoma | 3/3 | 5-fluorouracil | 3/3 | |
| Bahnson and Ratliff [41] | murine bladder carcinoma | 0/1 | actinomycin D | 1/1 | |
| Tiwari et al. [42] | human breast cancer | not assessed | tamoxifen | 1/1 | synergism was dose dependent |
| *TNF in combination with hyperthermia* | | | | | |
| Yamauchi et al. [43] | murine fibroblast-like carcinoma | 1/1 (TNF-α) | hyperthermia | 1/1 | |
| Tomasovic et al. [44] | murine fibroblast-like carcinoma | 1/1 (TNF-α)<br>1/1 (TNF-β)<br>1/1 (TNFsam2[2]) | hyperthermia | 1/1 (TNF-α)<br>1/1 (TNF-β)<br>1/1 (TNF-sam2) | optimal temperature: 39.0–40.5 °C/24 h; best results with TNF-β and TNF-sam2 |
| | murine mammary adenocarcinoma | 0/1 (TNF-α)<br>0/1 (TNF-β)<br>0/1 (TNF-sam2) | hyperthermia | 0/1<br>1/1<br>1/1 | best results with TNF-β and TNF-sam2, optimal temperature 43 °C for 1.5 h |
| | human bladder carcinoma | 0/1 (TNF-α)<br>0/1 (TNF-β)<br>0/1 (TNF-sam2) | hyperthermia | 0/0<br>0/0<br>0/0 | |

GM-CSF = Granulocyte-macrophage colony-stimulating factor.

1 Number with antiproliferative effect/number of cell lines investigated.

2 Recombinant molecule prepared by Soma et al. [45].

respond to some cytokines. TNF can cause myeloid differentiation in myeloid cell lines [25]. The effect of TNF on bone marrow aspirates from patients with acute or chronic myelogenous leukemia has been determined. A significant inhibitory effect on acute myeloid leukemia blast cells has been demonstrated. In chronic myelocytic leukemia (accelerated phase or blast crisis) an effect is also present [26].

### In vivo Antitumor Effects

Many studies have demonstrated that cytokine therapy prolongs survival of tumor-bearing mice, but partial and complete remission as defined in clinical studies may not be seen, or can only be assessed at postmortem examination. The meth A sarcoma was one of the first tumors studied [4]. This tumor shows the classical response with hemorrhagic necrosis after application of TNF. The antitumor effect of TNF was dose dependent, with greater activity at higher doses, with increased frequency of administration of TNF, and with intratumoral (i.t.) injection [46]. Only a small number of tumor cell lines were studied up to 1989. Many of them behave as highly malignant tumors. This makes them poor models for those tumors which are responsive to cytokine therapy in clinical practice [47]. From 1989 to 1992 more tumor cell lines have been studied.

*TNF Alone and in Combination with Other Cytokines*

TNF mediates the vasculotoxic effects of flavone acetic acid for sponge-implanted murine Colo 26 tumors [48]. Kallinowski et al. [49] studied the effect of TNF on tumor blood flow, oxygen consumption, and growth of a rat carcinosarcoma (DS carcinosarcoma). The changes in growth of subcutaneous DS carcinosarcoma tumors were dose dependent, and reflected in changes in tumor blood flow. Low TNF doses increased, but higher TNF doses inhibited tumor growth and tumor blood flow. Mice bearing a single B16 melanoma liver nodule were treated with TNF and TNF + IL-2 given with or without anti-B 16 monoclonal antibody. TNF administration augmented the antitumor effect of specific anti-B16 antibodies, and the addition of IL-2 further increased this antitumor effect [33]. TNF leads to a measurable tumor regression of transplanted cervical adenocarcinoma in nude mice [27]. RG-2 glioma cells without TNF-α receptors respond to neither intravenous (i.v.) administration nor to i.t. delivery of TNF-α [50]. The antitumor activity of TNF against subcutaneously (s.c.) implanted adenocarcinoma 755 in mice was enhanced by IL-2 [51]. Human renal cell carcinoma transplanted into nude mice was treated with TNF-α and/or IFN-α. All treatments resulted in a significantly reduced tumor growth. TNF-α plus IFN-α showed the greatest effect [52]. I.v. administration of TNF-α to nude mice bearing human prostate cancer resulted in significant inhibition of primary tumor growth; the growth of intra-abdominal PC3 tumors induced by intrasplenic injection of PC3 was also reduced. Complete remissions were not seen. The incidence of microscopic PC3 foci in the spleen, liver, lung, and diaphragm was diminished in mice receiving TNF therapy [29]. No effect was seen by cytokine combinations with TNF against Lewis lung carcinoma [51]. Mice bearing Lewis lung carcinoma showed a decrease in the number of pulmonary metastatic tumors when IL-1β was administered in combination with recombinant human (rh) TNF-α daily i.v., much more than when IL-1β was administered alone [53]. Inhibition of the development of experimental M109 lung metastases in mice was effective in >60% by intraperitoneal (i.p.) treatment with recombinant murine TNF-α [54].

*TNF in Combination with Cytotoxic Agents*

An increased antitumor effect against subcutaneous melanoma B16 tumors in mice with a combination of rhTNF-α and the microtubule effector DHPN, a fluorenone-azomethine derivate, has been observed [55]. Both BCNU (carmustine) and TNF caused tumor growth delay of B16 melanoma and of human melanoma xenografts in immune-deprived mice. The combination of low-dose TNF with BCNU resulted in significant growth delay in B16 melanoma; human melanoma xenografts yielded similar results but only at higher doses of TNF [56]. The combination of surgery and adjuvant or neoadjuvant rhTNF/etoposide therapy in A/J mice bearing the C1300 murine neuroblastoma appears to significantly delay the progression of disease. Neoadjuvant chemoimmunotherapy prior to surgical excision seems to prevent local disease recurrence and distant metastases [57]. Hyperthermia (43.5 °C) plus TNF i.v. in the treatment of experimental bladder carcinoma KK-47 in athymic mice showed significantly increased antitumor effects compared with hyperthermia alone [58]. Against androgen-dependent and -independent Dunning rat prostatic tumors combinations of IFN-γ and TNF had synergistic antiproliferative effects against all four tumor lines. Complete growth inhibitions could not be achieved, but survival was significantly increased [59]. Human colon cancer in nude mice was treated with rTNF-α and/or adriamycin entrapped in liposomes. Tumor growth inhibition was seen in all groups, the greatest therapeutic effect being observed with adriamycin after pretreatment with rTNF-α [60].

*TNF in Combination with Radiation*

TNF in combination with radiation caused an increase in the fraction of hypoxic cells in the murine KHT sarcoma [61].

*Intraperitoneal TNF*

In human gastric cancer tissues xenografted into nude mice, a suppression of tumor growth was observed when rhTNF was given i.p. in combination with hyperthermia at 43.5 °C. The tumoral blood flow decreased immediately after hyperthermia or rhTNF alone, or hyperthermia plus rhTNF. rhTNF alone was not effective [62].

Intraperitoneal injection of rhTNF in three i.p. nude mouse xenograft models of human ovarian cancer promoted micrometastatic peritoneal implants of tumor in all three xenograft models. The tumor burden of TNF-treated mice was smaller or equal compared to rhIL-1β-treated mice. TNF increased the survival of tumor-bearing mice [63].

*Intratumoral or Locoregional Treatment with TNF*

In the mouse bladder tumor model, MTB-2, intravesical treatment with TNF alone together with actinomycin D showed no significant results [41]. In a new nonimmunogenic rat bladder tumor model, RBT323, TNF showed dose-dependent and in combination with IFN-γ synergistic growth-inhibiting effects by administration peritumorally, and prolonged the time to tumor recurrence [64].

In a rat model for colon adenocarcinoma, tumor fragments implanted subcutaneously or under the hepatic capsule were treated with TNF i.v. or i.t. Equal doses were lethal when given i.v., but injection i.t. resulted in inhibition of tumor growth in the s.c. as well as subhepatic tumor model [65].

Human digestive-organ cancer xenografts transplanted in nude mice have been treated with rTNF alone or in combination with other biological-response modifiers. Esophageal cancer was most sensitive, while pancreatic, colonic, and gastric cancer were relatively sensitive to rTNF. All combinations of rTNF and other biological-response modifiers were more effective than rTNF alone. Gastric tumors completely regressed after treatment with a combination of rTNF and rIFN-γ or rTNF and picibanil (OK-432) [66].

## Clinical Experiences

### *Phase I Trials*

A large number of phase I trials have been performed with human TNF. Many different schedules and routes of administration have been studied in patients with advanced malignant diseases. The results of the years to 1989 have been reviewed by several authors [67, 68]. The phase I studies published between 1990 and 1992 are listed in table 3. Few responses in patients with several malignancies were reported. While phase I trials are designed only to determine toxicity, evidence of antitumor effects of rhTNF has been sought. Results have been disappointing: an overall response rate with rhTNF monotherapy in clinical trials from 1987–1989 of 4% was evaluated by Alexander and Rosenberg [67] and Spriggs and Yates [68]. In clinial phase I trials with rhTNF alone and in combination with cytokines from 1990–1992 similar response rates were observed. The common toxicities are described below.

*Systemic Toxicities*

Side effects include fever, chills and rigors, myalgias, nausea, vomiting and fatigue. Rigors after TNF administration are common, but not observed by all investigators [70, 73]. Fever follows generally rapidly after i.v. infusion of TNF [69, 70, 72, 79] and also occurs after i.t. administration [73]. Antipyretic drugs can ameliorate fever, especially when they are given before TNF infusion; an effect on rigor has not be seen [67, 73]. Myalgias and fatigue occur in most patients, nausea and vomiting in 20–40%. After administration of TNF into skin, soft tissue, or muscle, local effects are seen, which are in some cases dose limiting [67, 72].

*Hemodynamic Effects*

After i.v. bolus administration, short hypertension, associated with rising temperatures and rigor can be observed in 10–20% of patients. Acute pulmonary edema can also occur in rare cases; the mechanism is not yet clear [81]. 2–12 h after TNF i.v. administration, hypotension regularly occurs; this major side effect was dose limiting in most phase I trials. Adequate prehydratation may help to ameliorate hypotension [67, 68].

*Hepatotoxicity*

Transient alterations in serum transaminases are commonly observed following TNF infusions [68, 69, 79, 82–85]. The increase of serum glutamic-oxaloacetic transami-

**Table 3.** Phase I studies in patients with advanced malignancies

| Author | Histology[1] | Administration | Dose μg/m² | n | Dose-limiting toxicity | Effect[2] |
|---|---|---|---|---|---|---|
| *Intravenous bolus or short-infusion administration* | | | | | | |
| Gamm et al. [69] | colon, renal, multiple myeloma, sarcoma, acute/chronic leukemia, pancreas | 30 min infusion twice days 1–5 every 2nd week | 5–400 | 62 | hypotension, hepatotoxicity | PR colon cancer (1) pancreatic carcinoma (1) CLL (1) |
| Schiller et al. [71] | colon, renal, gastrointestinal, lung | 30 min infusion 3 times weekly | 2–275 | 53 | hypotension, fatigue, nausea | PR colon cancer (1) |
| Krigel et al. [71] | colon, pancreas | 15 min infusion days 1, 8–12 | 160 | 27 | hypotension, hemorrhagic gastritis | none |
| *Intramuscular or subcutaneous administration* | | | | | | |
| Aulitzki et al. [72] | hepatocellular carcinoma, colon, melanoma, sarcoma | s.c. or i.m. twice weekly | 1–100 | 17 | fever, hypotension, severe local reaction | NC in 1 patient with hepatocellular carcinoma |
| *Intratumoral administration* | | | | | | |
| Ijzermans et al. [73] | liver metastases from colon, pancreas, bile duct, adenocarcinoma | single i.t. bolus every 4 weeks | 100–250[3] | 12 | fever, chill | none |
| *Hepatic arterial infusion* | | | | | | |
| Mavligit et al. [74] | liver metastasis from colon, leiomyosarcoma, melanoma | hepatic arterial infusion for 5 days | 12,5–175 | 22 | hypophosphatemia | PR (2 patients) MR (3 patients) |
| *Intraperitoneal administration* | | | | | | |
| Hardy et al. [75] | ovarian cancer | i.p. once every 4 weeks | 89 | 4 | | none |
| Räth et al. [76] | ovarian adenocarcinoma | i.p. once weekly for 2 months | 40–350 | 29 | | CR + PR in 76% |
| Werner et al. [77] | ascites in gynecological cancer | i.p. up to 3 times every 2–3 weeks | 8 | 8 | | response in 87.5% |
| *Combination with other cytokines* | | | | | | |
| Schiller et al. [78] | colon, renal, melanoma | IFN-γ and TNF: 30 min infusion 3 times weekly | 25–100 IFN: 100 | 24 | hypotension | none |
| Yang et al. [79] | non-small cell lung cancer | daily IL-2 $6 \times 10^6$ IU/m², and TNF i.m. × 5 every 3 weeks | 25–100 | 16 | fever, local reaction, pancytopenia | PR: adeno-carcinoma (1); MR: adeno- (2) + squamous cell carcinoma (1) |
| Negrier et al. [80] | renal, melanoma, breast, colon | IL-2 $18 \times 10^6$ IU/m² × 6 and TNF × 3 per day at day 7 | 10–120/day | 34 | pulmonary toxicity | PR breast cancer (1) renal cancer (1) |

PR = Partial response; CLL = chronic lymphocytic leukemia; NC = no change; MR = minor response; CR = complete response.

1 Histology and site shown are the most frequent for each series.

2 Number of patients given in parentheses.

3 Total dose.

nase is usually higher than the increase of serum glutamic-pyruvic transaminase, alkaline phosphatase, or bilirubin. Schedules with administration of TNF twice daily are more hepatotoxic [69].

*Nephrotoxicity*
After infusion of TNF, a decrease in urine output is common. Transient, reversible elevations of blood urea nitrogen and creatinine have been reported, although this has not been found in all studies [79].

*Pulmonary Toxicity*
Pulmonary toxicity consisting of decreased lung diffusion capacity has been reported [86]. Anaphylactic-like reactions, bronchospasms, and adult respiratory distress syndrome were seen in several patients immediately after rTNF infusions following a 6-day treatment with IL-2, irrespective of the rTNF dose or treatment cycle, and mainly in patiens with extensive pulmonary metastases [80].

*Hematological Toxicity*
TNF has only weak effects on peripheral blood cell counts. Granulocytes are decreased in most reports of 5-day schedules; a transient drop of granulocytes, monocytes and lymphocytes has also been observed during TNF infusion; recovery of monocytes and lymphocytes was more prolonged. A slight decrease in platelet counts was seen in 24-hour infusion schedules and in 5-day administration schedules. Anemia and thrombocytopenia can occur, but do not generally limit the administration of TNF [68, 69, 87, 88].

*Effects on Coagulation*
Disseminated intravascular coagulopathy may occur and it has caused pulmonary emboli [89]. Alterations in prothrombin time and partial thromboplastin time were transient. In several patients with pancreatic or gastric carcinoma deep venous thrombosis appeared [81]. Retinal vein thrombosis [84] and intracranial hemorrhage [81] have also been observed.

*Neurotoxicity*
A common toxicity associated with TNF administration is headache. Lethargy and fatigue are also frequently observed. Transient amnesia, aphasia, hallucination and diplopia have all been reported [67–70, 85].

*Effects on Metabolism*
After administration of TNF i.v. or as an intramuscular injection, cholesterol and high-density lipoproteins are significantly decreased, while triglycerides and very-low-density lipoproteins are increased [68].

*Other Toxicity*
Hypophosphatemia, probably resulting from an intracellular shift of phosphate, associated with clinically significant, right-sided myocardial dysfunction and severe lassitude have been observed. These side effects were promptly reversed after rTNF was stopped and intravenous phosphate supplementation was started [90]. One case of pulmonary hemorrhage has been reported [82]. Repeated TNF infusion may lead to a permanent decrease in myocardial contractility and, ultimately, congestive cardiomyopathy [91]. Hemorrhagic gastritis has been observed in only one phase I trial, in 11% of patients [71].

## *Phase II Trials*

In phase I trials with human TNF alone or in combination, responses were rare. This is not surprising, because phase I trials are designed only to evaluate toxicity. Patients have mostly resistant tumors and have received prior therapy. Several well-designed phase II trials have been performed, but few responses to TNF therapy have been reported. An overview is shown in table 4, 5.

*Responses*
In colorectal carcinoma, one partial response was seen in a patient with local recurrence of a rectum primary tumor and liver metastasis treated with 130 μg/m$^2$ for 3 days every second week [83]. In another trial, TNF was given on days 1, 3 and 5 with dose escalation from 217 to 652 μg/m$^2$. One minor response was seen in a patient, with disappearance of retroperitoneal lymph nodes [92].

In a trial of the Southwest Oncology Group [81] of TNF in bladder cancer, one partial remission has been seen. Skillings et al. [85] treated 26 patients with renal cell carcinoma with 150 μg/m$^2$ TNF i.v. for 5 consecutive days. One complete response in a patient with contralateral kidney and one lung metastasis, and one partial response of a primary kidney lesion, with complete regression of lung nodules, and improved bone scan were reported. In an abstract, a response rate of 4/22 patients in combined therapy with TNF-α 50–100 μg/m$^2$ administered as a 24-hour infusion once a week and IFN-γ in

**Table 4.** Phase II trials of human TNF i.v. administration

| Author | Cancer | Administration | Dose μg/m² | n | Responses per number evaluable |
|---|---|---|---|---|---|
| Heim et al. [83] | colon | i.v. day 1–3 every 2nd week | 130 | 15 | 1/11 (1 PR) |
| Schaadt et al. [92] | colon | i.v. days 1, 3, 5 every 4th week | 217–652 | 15 | 0/15 (1 MR) |
| Kemeny et al. [84] | colon | i.v. twice days 1–5 every 2nd week | 100–150 | 16 | 0/14 |
| Whitehead et al. [87] | colon | i.v. days 1–5 every 2nd week | 150 | 25 | 0/22 |
| Brown et al. [89] | pancreas | i.v. days 1–5 every 2nd week | 150 | 26 | 0/22 |
| Hersh et al. [81] | stomach | i.v. days 1–5 every 2nd week | 150 | 29 | 0/26 |
| Budd et al. [93] | breast | i.v. days 1–5 every 2nd week | 150 | 22 | 0/19 |
| Hersh et al. [81] | renal | i.v. days 1–5 every 2nd week | 150 | 10 | 1/9 (1 PR) |
| Skillings et al. [85] | renal | i.v. days 1–5 every 2nd week | 150 | 26 | 2/22 (1 CR, 1 PR) |
| Hersh et al. [81] | endometrium | i.v. days 1–5 every 2nd week | 150 | 5 | 0/3 |
| Hersh et al. [81] | myleoma | i.v. days 1–5 every 2nd week | 150 | 9 | 0/9 |
| Rinehart et al. [94] | sarcoma | i.v. days 1–5 every 2nd week | 150 | 21 | 0/18 |

CR = Complete response; PR = partial response; MR = minor response.

**Table 5.** Phase II trials of human TNF in combination with IFN

| Author | Cancer | Administration | Dose μg/m² | n | Responses per number evaluable |
|---|---|---|---|---|---|
| Fiedler et al. [95] | colon | TNF i.v. day 1–5 weekly | 50 | 16 | 0/14 |
| | | IFN-γ s.c. day 1–5 weekly | 0.1 mg | | |
| Sohn et al. [96] | renal | TNF i.v./24 h weekly | 160 | 14 | 4/22 (CR or PR) |
| | | IFN-γ 3 × /week | $18 \times 10^6$ U | | |
| Abbruzzese et al. [97] | colon | | | 7 | * |
| | pancreas | TNF i.v. day 1–5 | 125 | 4 | |
| | bile duct | IFN-γ s.c. day 1–5 | 125 | 2 | |

* Trial has been terminated because of excessive toxicity.

renal cell carcinoma was reported by Sohn et al. [96]. A case report of a partial remission of a hepatocellular carcinoma has been reported by Maeda et al. [98]. The patient was treated with TNF once a week together with local hyperthermia.

*Local Administration of TNF*

*Intraperitoneal Therapy.* With instillation of drugs into the peritoneal cavity, high local drug concentrations are achievable. The promising results of phase I trials with TNF i.p. in gynecological malignancies [76, 77] were confirmed in phase II trials [99]. Complete resolution of ascites has been observed in 17 of 32 patients with TNF 80 μg/m² weekly. 14 others had more than a 50% decrease in ascites. The solid tumor mass was not affected. With a combination therapy of TNF and IFN-α or IFN-γ, a response in solid tumors with a size <0.2 cm and a response in ascites was seen [100].

*Intra-Arterial Treatment of Brain Tumors.* In a Japanese phase II trial, 20 patients with malignant glioma were treated with intra-arterial injections of TNF. Optimal doses were $1 \times 10^5$ U/m²/day. The treatment was repeated 3–9 times at 7- to 14-day intervals. Complete response was seen in 1 patient, partial response in 2 patients, while another 4 patients had documented tumor necrosis [101].

*Isolation Perfusion of Limb.* In an ongoing study, Liénard et al. [102] treated 29 patients with multiple progressive in transit melanoma metastases of the lower limb (stage IIIa or IIIab). rTNF-α at the unique dose of 4 mg was injected as a bolus in the arterial line, under mild hyperthermic conditions (40–40.5 °C) for 90 min. rIFN-γ was given s.c. on days –2 and –1, and in the perfusate with rTNF-α at the dose of 0.2 mg. Melphalan was administered in the perfusate at a dose giving a concentration of 40 μg/ml. In 90%, complete responses, and in 10%, partial responses have been observed. Since then, 49 patients have been reported. 27 had recurrences after this isolated limb perfusion. The response rate remained 90% complete response and 10% partial response [103]. In another publication, 3 patients with sarcoma and 1 patient with malignant fibrohistiocytoma are additionally reported. Three patients responded completely, the other partially [104]. Hypotension, fever, adult respiratory distress syndrome, bilirubin elevation, neutropenia grade 3 (1 case) and grade 4 (1 case), and thrombocytopenia grade 4 (1 case) occurred. Another abstract reports treatment of 19 patients with soft-tissue sarcoma, with a complete response in 7 and a partial response in 9 patients [105].

## Future Aspects

Although TNF is an effective agent in vitro and in some experimental tumor models, few responses are obtained with systemic application of TNF as a single agent. Dose appears to be an important determinant of response, but is limited by toxicity. Combination trials with IFNs and other cytotoxic agents have started, but have not yet shown promising results. Further investigations to evaluate responses in combination therapy are necessary. Interventions to decrease TNF side effects, and better patient selection to exclude TNF-resistant patients must be integrated into study designs. More promising results than the above-mentioned ones are reported for local administration of TNF.

Phase II trials with i.p. administration of TNF showed a reduction of malignant ascites in more than 85%. Combination with IFN-α or IFN-γ may cause tumor regression of small i.p. tumors. The results with intra-arterial therapy of malignant glioma and liver metastasis are very encouraging and need to be pursued. The results of isolation limb perfusion with high-dose TNF-α in combination with IFN-γ and melphalan in melanoma and sarcoma performed by Liénard et al. [102–104] must be emphasized because of their outstandingly high response rates. These results suggest that future investigational efforts of TNF administration in the treatment of malignancies should be aimed at local treatment. It seems unlikely that TNF will play a significant role as a systemic therapy for human cancer.

## References


1 Balkwill FR, Naylor MS, Malik S: Tumour necrosis factor as an anticancer agent. Eur J Cancer 1990;26:641–644.
2 Coley Nauts H, Fowler GA, Bogatko FH: A review of the influence of bacterial infections and of bacterial products (Coley's toxins) on malignant tumors in man. Acta Med Scand Suppl 1953;274:29–97.
3 Shear MJ, Perrault A: Chemical treatment of tumors. IX. Reactions of mice with primary subcutaneous tumors to injection of a hemorrhage-producing bacterial polysaccharide. J Natl Cancer Inst 1944;44:461–476.
4 Carswell EA, Old LJ, Kassel RJ, Green S, Fiore N, Williamson B: An endotoxin-induced serum factor which causes necrosis of tumors. Proc Natl Acad Sci USA 1975;72:3666–3670.
5 Matthews N: Tumor necrosis factor from the rabbit. V. Synthesis in vitro by mononuclear phagocytes from various tissues of normal and BCG injected rabbits. Br J Cancer 1980;44: 418–424.
6 Matthews N: Production of an antitumour cytotoxin by human monocytes. Immunology 1981;44:135–142.
7 Aggarwal BB, Kohr WJ, Hass PE, Moffat B, Spencer SA, Henzel WJ, Bringman TS, Nedwin GE, Goeddel DV, Harkins RN: Human tumor necrosis factor. Production, purification, and characterization. J Biol Chem 1985; 260:2345–2354.
8 Beutler B, Mahoney J, Le-Trang N, Pekala P, Cerami A: Purification of cachectin, a lipoprotein lipase-suppressing hormone secreted by endotoxin-induced RAW 264.7 cells. J Exp Med 1985;161:984–995.
9 Beutler B, Greenwald D, Hulmes JD, Chang M, Pan YC, Mathison J, Ulevitch R, Cerami A: Identity of tumor necrosis factor and the macrophage-secreted factor cachectin. Nature 1985;316:552–554.
10 Aggarwal BB, Moffat B, Harkins RN: Human lymphotoxin: Production by a lymphoblastoid line, purification, and initial characterization. J Biol Chem 1984;259:686–691.
11 Nedwin GE, Naylor SL, Sakaguchi AY, Smith D, Jarrett-Nedwin J, Pennica D, Goeddel DV, Gray PW: Human lymphotoxin and tumor necrosis factor genes: Structure, homology and chromosomal localization. Nucleic Acids Res 1985;13:6361–6373.
12 Aggarwal BB: Structure of tumor necrosis factor and its receptor. Biotherapy 1991;3:113–120.
13 Hohmann HP, Remy R, Brockhaus M, van Loon APGM: Two different cell types have different major receptors for human tumor necrosis factor (TNF alpha). J Biol Chem 1989;264: 14927–14934.
14 Brockhaus M, Schoenfeld HJ, Schlaeger EJ, Hunziker W, Lesslauer W, Loetscher H: Identification of two types of tumor necrosis factor receptors on human cell lines by monoclonal antibodies. Proc Natl Acad Sci USA 1990;87: 3127–3131.
15 Schall TJ, Lewis M, Koller KJ, Lee A, Rice GC, Wong GH, Gatanaga T, Granger GA, Lentz R, Raab H, Kohr WJ, Goeddel DV: Molecular cloning and expression of a receptor for human tumor necrosis factor. Cell 1990;61:361–370.
16 Loetscher H, Pan YC, Lahm HW, Gentz R, Brockhaus M, Tabuchi H, Lesslauer W: Molecular cloning and expression of the human 55 kDa tumor necrosis factor receptor. Cell 1990; 61:351–359.

17 Smith C, Davis T, Anderson D, Solam L, Beckmann MP, Jerzy R, Dower SK, Cosman D, Goodwin RG: A receptor for tumor necrosis factor defines an unusual family of cellular and viral proteins. Science 1990;248:1019–1023.
18 Aggarwal BB, Eessalu TE: Induction of receptors for tumour necrosis factor-alpha by interferons is not a major mechanism for their synergistic cytotoxic response. J Biol Chem 1987;262:10000–10007.
19 Aggarwal BB, Eessalu TE: Effect of phorbol esters on down-regulation and redistribution of cell surface receptors for tumor necrosis factor-alpha. J Biol Chem 1987;262:16450–16455.
20 Holtmann H, Wallach D: Down regulation of the receptors for tumor necrosis factor by interleukin 1 and 4 beta-phorbol-12-myristate-13-acetate. J Immunol 1987;139:1161–1167.
21 Ding AH, Sanchez E, Srimal S, Nathan CF: Macrophages rapidly internalize their tumor necrosis factor receptors in response to bacterial lipopolysaccharide. J Biol Chem 1989;264: 3924–3929.
22 Johnson SE, Baglioni C: Tumor necrosis factor receptors and cytocidal activity are down-regulated by activators of protein kinase C. J Biol Chem 1988;263:5686–5692.
23 Spriggs DR: Tumor necrosis factor: Basic principles and preclinical studies; in DeVita VT Jr, Hellman S, Rosenberg SA (eds): Biologic Therapy of Cancer. Philadelphia, Lippincott, 1991, pp 354–377.
24 Giaccone G, Kadoyama C, Maneckjee R, Venzon D, Alexander RB, Gazdar AF: Effects of tumor necrosis factor, alone or in combination with topoisomerase-II-targeted drugs, on human lung cancer cell lines. Int J Cancer 1990; 46:326–329.
25 Jones AL, Selby P: Clinical applications of tumour necrosis factor. Prog Growth Factor Res 1989;1:107–122.
26 Kleine HD, Wagner U, Poliwoda H, Freund M: Effects of tumour necrosis factor α on bone marrow aspirates of patients with acute myelogeneous leukemia determined by flow-cytometric cell-cycle analysis. J Cancer Res Clin Oncol 1992;118:56–60.
27 Iwasaka T, Hara K, Hayashi Y, Yokoyama M, Hachisuga T, Fukuda K, Okuma Y, Sugimori H: Antitumor effects of human recombinant interferon-gamma and tumor necrosis factor on five cervical adenocarcinoma cell lines, in vivo and in vitro. Gynecol Oncol 1991;42:39–43.
28 van de Loosdrecht AA, Ossenkoppele GJ, Beelen RH, Broekhoven MG, Langenhuijsen MM: Role of interferon gamma and tumour necrosis factor alpha in monocyte-mediated cytostasis and cytotoxicity against a human histiocytic lymphoma cell line. Cancer Immunol Immunother 1992;34:393–398.
29 Sherwood ER, Ford TR, Lee C, Kozlowski JM: Therapeutic efficacy of recombinant tumor necrosis factor alpha in an experimental model of human prostatic carcinoma. J Biol Response Modif 1990;9:44–52.
30 Hand AM, Husgafvel Pursiainen K, Temmilehto L, Mattson K, Linnainmaa K: Malignant mesothelioma: The antiproliferative effect of cytokine combinations on three human mesothelioma cell lines. Cancer Lett 1991;58:205–210.
31 Bowman RV, Manning LS, Davis MR, Robinson BW: Chemosensitivity and cytokine sensitivity of malignant mesothelioma. Cancer Chemother Pharmacol 1991;28:420–426.
32 Denis M, Ghadirian E: Human monocyte tumouristatic ability: Modulation by cytokines and tumour cell products. Int J Immunopharmacol 1990;12:509–513.
33 Eisenthal A, McIntosh JK: Effect of recombinant human tumour necrosis factor alpha on the induction of antibody-dependent cellular cytotoxicity in the treatment of established B16 melanoma liver nodules. Cancer Immunol Immunother 1990;31:243–249.
34 Raitano AB, Scuderi P, Korc M: Binding and biological effects of tumor necrosis factor and gamma interferon in human pancreatic carcinoma cells. Pancreas 1990;5:267–277.
35 Sacchi M, Klapan I, Johnson JT, Whiteside TL: Antiproliferative effects of cytokines on squamous cell carcinoma. Arch Otolaryngol Head Neck Surg 1991;117:321–326.
36 Massad LS, Mutch DG, Kao MS, Powell CB, Collins JL: Inhibition of protein synthesis enhances the lytic effects of tumor necrosis factor alpha and interferon gamma in cell lines derived from gynecological malignancies. Cancer Immunol Immunother 1991;33:183–188.
37 Hoon DS, Okun E, Banez M, Irie RF, Morton DL: Interleukin 4 alone and with gamma-interferon or alpha-tumor necrosis factor inhibits cell growth and modulates cell surface antigens on human renal cell carcinomas. Cancer Res 1991;51:5687–5693.
38 Bonavida B, Tsuchitani T, Zighelboim J, Berek JS: Synergy is documented in vitro with low-dose recombinant tumor necrosis factor, cisplatin, and doxorubicin in ovarian cancer cells. Gynecol Oncol 1990;38:333–339.
39 Vigani A, Chiara S, Miglietta L, Repetto L, Conte PF, Cimoli G, Morelli L, Billi G, Parodi S, Russo P: Effect of recombinant human tumor necrosis factor on A2774 human ovarian cancer cell line: Potentiation of mitoxantrone cytotoxicity. Gynecol Oncol 1991;41:52–55.
40 Schiller JH, Bittner G: Anti-proliferative effects of tumor necrosis factor, gamma interferon and 5-fluorouracil on human colorectal carcinoma cell lines. Int J Cancer 1990;46:61–66.
41 Bahnson RR, Ratliff TL: In vitro and in vivo anti-tumor activity of recombinant mouse tumour necrosis factor (TNF) in a mouse bladder tumor (MBT-2). J Urol 1990;144:172–175.
42 Tiwari RK, Wong GY, Liu J, Miller D, Osborne MP: Augmentation of cytotoxicity using combinations of interferons (types I and II), tumor necrosis factor-alpha, and tamoxifen in MCF-7 cells. Cancer Lett 1991;61:45–52.
43 Yamauchi N, Watanabe N, Maeda M, Okamoto T, Sasaki H, Tsuji N, Tsuji Y, Umeno H, Akiyama S, Niitsu Y: Mechanism of synergistic cytotoxic effect between tumor necrosis factor and hyperthermia. Jpn J Cancer Res 1992;83: 540–545.
44 Tomasovic SP, Lu S, Klostergaard J: Comparative in vitro studies of the potentiation of tumor necrosis factor (TNF)-α, TNF-β, and TNF-SAM2 cytotoxicity by hyperthermia. J Immunother 1992;11:85–92.
45 Soma G, Tsuji Y, Tanabe Y, Noguchi K, Kitahara Tanabe N, Gatanaga T, Inagawa H, Kawakami M, Mizuno D: Biological activities of novel recombinant tumor necrosis factor having N-terminal amino acid sequences derived from cytotoxic factors produced by THP-1 cells. J Biol Response Modif 1988;7:587–595.
46 Malik STA: The activity of TNF in experimental cancer models; in Beutler B (ed): Tumor Necrosis Factors: The Molecules and Their Emerging Role in Medicine. New York, Raven, 1992, pp 407–423.
47 Thomas H, Balkwill FR: Effects of interferons and other cytokines on tumors in animals: A review. Pharmacol Ther 1991;52:307–330.
48 Madhevan V, Malik STA, Maeger T, Fiers W, Hart I: Role of tumor necrosis factor in flavone acetic acid-induced tumor vascular shutdown. Cancer Res 1990;50:5537–5542.
49 Kallinowski F, Moehle R, Schaefer C, Vaupel P: Effects of tumor necrosis factor-alpha on tumor blood flow and hyperthermic treatment. Onkologie 1989;12:131–135.
50 Kiwit JC, Schmitz KH, Daum L, Reifenberger G, Roosen N: Effects of recombinant human tumor necrosis factor on rodent gliomas and normal brain. J Neurosurg 1991;75:597–603.
51 Iigo M, Nishikata K, Hoshi A: Effect of recombinant interleukin-1 alpha, recombinant interleukin-2, recombinant interferon-beta, and recombinant tumor necrosis factor on subcutaneously implanted adenocarcinoma 755 and Lewis lung carcinoma. J Biol Response Modif 1990;9:426–430.
52 Baisch H, Otto U, Klöppel G: Antiproliferative and cytotoxic effects of single and combined treatment with tumor necrosis factor alpha and/or alpha interferon on a human renal cell carcinoma xenotransplanted into nu/nu mice: Cell kinetic studies. Cancer Res 1990;50:6389–6395.
53 Ohkura M, Fuchimoto S, Orita K: Antitumor effect of recombinant human interleukin-1 beta alone and in combination with natural human tumor necrosis factor-alpha. Jpn J Cancer Res 1990;81:1026–1031.
54 Schultz RM, Altom MG: Protective activity of recombinant murine tumor necrosis factor-alpha and interferon-gamma against experimental murine lung carcinoma metastases. J Interferon Res 1990;10:229–236.
55 Jones AL, Millar JL, Millar BC, Powell B, Selby P, Winkley A, Lakhani S, Gore ME, McElwain TJ: Enhanced anti-tumor activity of carmustine (BCNU) with tumour necrosis factor in vitro and vivo. Br J Cancer 1990;62:776–780.

56 Baumgart J, Schlott B, Suehnel J, Vater W, Schulze W, Behnke D: Synergistic cytotoxicity of human recombinant tumour necrosis factor alpha combined with microtubule effectors. J Cancer Res Clin Oncol 1991;117:239–243.
57 Leonard MP, Gearhart JP, Jeffs RD: Chemoimmunotherapy in conjunction with surgery: Strategies for management of murine neuroblastoma. J Pediatr Surg 1991;26:1224–1229.
58 Amano T, Kumini K, Nakashima K, Uchibayashi T, Hisazumi H: A combined therapy of hyperthermia and tumor necrosis factor for nude mice bearing KK-47 bladder cancer. J Urol 1990;144:370–374.
59 van Moorselaar RJ, Hendriks BT, van Stratum P, van der Meide PH, Debruyne FM, Schalken JA: Synergistic antitumor effects of rat gamma-interferon and human tumor necrosis factor alpha against androgen-dependent and- independent rat prostatic tumors. Cancer Res 1991; 51:2329–2334.
60 Maruo Y, Konno H, Baba S: Therapeutic effects of liposomal adriamycin in combination with tumor necrosis factor-alpha. J Surg Oncol 1992;49:20–24.
61 Edwards HS, Bremner JC, Stratford IJ: Induction of hypoxia in the KHT sarcoma by tumour necrosis factor and flavone acetic acid. Int J Radiat Biol 1991;59:419–432.
62 Fujimoto S, Konno C, Kobayashi K, Kokubun M, Shrestha RD, Kiuchi S, Takahashi M, Ohta M, Okui K: Augmented antitumour effects of combined treatment with hyperthermia and tumour necrosis factor on human gastric cancer xenotransplanted into nude mice. Int J Hyperthermia 1991;7:511–518.
63 Malik ST, East N, Boraschi D, Balkwill FR: Effects of intraperitoneal recombinant interleukin-1 beta in intraperitoneal human ovarian cancer xenograft models: Comparison with the effects of tumour necrosis factor. Br J Cancer 1992;65:661–666.
64 van Moorselaar RJ, Hendriks BT, Borm G, van der Meide PH, Debruyne FM, Schalken JA: Inhibition of rat bladder tumor (RBT323) growth by tumor necrosis factor alpha and interferon-gamma in vivo. J Urol 1992;148: 458–462.
65 Ijzermans JN, Scheringa M, van der Schelling GP, Geerling RA, Marquet RL, Jeekel J: Injection of recombinant tumor necrosis factor directly into liver metastases: An experimental and clinical approach. Clin Exp Metastasis 1992;10:91–97.
66 Nio Y, Shiraishi T, Tsubono M, Morimoto H, Tseng CC, Kawabata K, Masai Y, Tun T, Fukumoto M, Tobe T: In vivo effects of human recombinant tumor necrosis factor alone and in combination with other biological response modifiers on human digestive organ cancer xenografts transplanted in nude mice. Biotherapy 1991;3:337–344.
67 Alexander RB, Rosenberg SA: Tumor necrosis factor: Clinical applications; in DeVita VT Jr, Hellman S, Rosenberg SA (eds): Biologic Therapy of Cancer. Philadelphia, Lippincott, 1991, pp 378–392.
68 Spriggs DR, Yates SW: Experiences with TNF administration in humans; in Beutler B (ed): Tumor Necrosis Factors: The Molecules and Their Emerging Role in Medicine. New York, Raven, 1992, pp 383–406.
69 Gamm H, Lindemann A, Mertelsmann R, Herrmann F: Phase 1 trial of recombinant human tumour necrosis factor alpha in patients with advanced malignancy. Eur J Cancer 1991; 27:856–863.
70 Schiller JH, Storer BE, Witt PL, Alberti D, Tombes MB, Arzoomanian R, Proctor RA, McCarthy D, Brown RR, Voss SD, Remick SC, Grem JL, Borden EC, Trump DL: Biological and clinical effects of intravenous tumor necrosis factor-alpha administered three times weekly. Cancer Res 1991;51:1651–1658.
71 Krigel RL, Padavic Shaller KA, Rudolph AA, Young JD, Weiner LM, Konrad M, Comis RL: Hemorrhagic gastritis as a new dose-limiting toxicity of recombinant tumor necrosis factor. J Natl Cancer Inst 1991;83:129–131.
72 Aulitzky WE, Tilg H, Gastl G, Mull R, Flener R, Vogel W, Herold M, Berger M, Judmaier G, Huber C: Recombinant tumour necrosis factor alpha administered subcutaneously or intramuscularly for treatment of advanced malignant disease: A phase I trial. Eur J Cancer 1991;27:462–467.
73 Ijzermans JN, Scheringa M, van der Schelling GP, Geerling RA, Marquet RL, Jeekel J: Injection of recombinant tumor necrosis factor directly into liver metastases: An experimental and clinical approach. Clin Exp Metastasis 1992;10:91–97.
74 Mavligit GM, Zukiwski AA, Charnsangavej C, Carrasco CH, Wallace S, Gutterman JU: Regional biologic therapy. Hepatic arterial infusion of recombinant human tumor necrosis factor in patients with liver metastases. Cancer 1992;69:557–561.
75 Hardy J, Jones A, Gore ME, Viner C, Selby P, Wiltshaw E: Treatment of advanced ovarian cancer with intraperitoneal tumour necrosis factor (letter). Eur J Cancer 1990;26:771.
76 Räth U, Kaufmann M, Schmid H, Hofmann J, Wiedenmann B, Kist A, Kempeni J, Schlick E, Bastert G, Kommerell B, Männel D: Effect of intraperitoneal recombinant human tumour necrosis factor alpha on malignant ascites. Eur J Cancer 1991;27:121–125.
77 Werner A, Mallmann P, Diedrich K, Wagner U, Krebs D: Lokoregionale Ascitestherapie mit Zytostatika und Immunmodulatoren bei gynäkologischen Malignomen. Zentralbl Gynäkol 1991;113:1313–1322.
78 Schiller JH, Witt PL, Storer B, Alberti D, Tombes MB, Arzoomanian R, Brown RR, Proctor RA, Voss SD, Spriggs DR, Trump DL, Border EC: Clinical and biologic effects of combination therapy with gamma interferon and tumor necrosis factor. Cancer 1992;69: 562–571.
79 Yang SC, Grimm EA, Parkinson DR, Carinhas J, Fry KD, Mendiguren Rodriguez A, Licciardello J, Owen Schaub LB, Hong WK, Roth JA: Clinical and immunomodulatory effects of combination immunotherapy with low-dose interleukin 2 and tumor necrosis factor alpha in patients with advanced non-small cell lung cancer: A phase I trial. Cancer Res 1991;51: 3669–3676.
80 Negrier MS, Pourreau CN, Palmer PA, Ranchere JY, Mercatello A, Viens P, Blaise D, Jasmin C, Misset JL, Franks CR, Maraninchi D, Philip T: Phase I trial of recombinant interleukin-2 followed by recombinant tumor necrosis factor in patients with metastatic cancer. J Immunother 1992;11:93–102.
81 Hersh EM, Metch BS, Muggia FM, Brown TD, Whitehead RP, Budd GT, Rinehart JJ, Crawford ED, Bonnet JD, Behrens BC: Phase II studies of recombinant human tumor necrosis factor alpha in patients with malignant disease: A summary of the Southwest Oncology Group experience. J Immunother 1991;10:426–431.
82 Schilling PJ, Murray JL, Markowitz AB: Novel tumor necrosis factor toxic effects. Pulmonary hemorrhage and severe hepatic dysfunction. Cancer 1992;69:256–260.
83 Heim ME, Siegmund R, Illiger HJ, Klee M, Rieche K, Berdel WE, Edler L: Tumor necrosis factor in advanced colorectal cancer: A phase II study. A trial of the phase I/II study group of the Association for Medical Oncology of the German Cancer Society. Onkologie 1990;13: 444–447.
84 Kemeny N, Childs B, Larchian W, Rosado K, Kelsen D: A phase II trial of recombinant tumor necrosis factor in patients with advanced colorectal carcinoma. Cancer 1990;66: 659–663.
85 Skillings J, Wierzbicki R, Eisenhauer E, Venner P, Letendre F, Stewart D, Weinerman B: A phase II study of recombinant tumor necrosis factor in renal cell carcinoma: A study of the National Cancer Institute of Canada Clinical Trials Group. J Immunother 1992;11:67–70.
86 Kuei JH, Tashkin DP, Figlin RA: Pulmonary toxicity of recombinant human tumor necrosis factor. Chest 1989;96:334–338.
87 Whitehead RP, Fleming T, Macdonald JS, Goodman PJ, Neefe J, Braun TJ, Swinnen LJ, Hersh EM: A phase II trial of recombinant tumor necrosis factor in patients with metastatic colorectal adenocarcinoma: A Southwest Oncology Group study. J Biol Response Modif 1990;9:588–591.
88 Aulitzky WE, Tilg H, Vogel W, Aulitzky W, Berger M, Gastl G, Herold M, Huber C: Acute hematologic effects of interferon alpha, interferon gamma, tumor necrosis factor alpha and interleukin 2. Ann Hematol 1991;62:25–31.
89 Brown TD, Goodman P, Fleming T, Macdonald JS, Hersh EM, Braun TJ: A phase II trial of recombinant tumor necrosis factor in patients with adenocarcinoma of the pancreas: A Southwest Oncology Group study. J Immunother 1991;10:376–378.

90 del Giglio A, Zukiwski AA, Ali MK, Mavligit GM: Severe, symptomatic, dose-limiting hypophosphatemia induced by hepatic arterial infusion of recombinant tumor necrosis factor in patients with liver metastases. Cancer 1991;67:2459–2461.
91 Hegewisch S, Weh HJ, Hossfeld DK: TNF-induced cardiomyopathy (letter). Lancet 1990;335:294–295.
92 Schaadt M, Pfreundschuh M, Lorscheidt G, Peters KM, Steinmetz T, Diehl V: Phase II study of recombinant human tumor necrosis factor in colorectal carcinoma. J Biol Response Modif 1990;9:247–250.
93 Budd GT, Green S, Baker LH, Hersh EP, Weick JK, Osborne CK: A Southwest Oncology Group phase II trial of recombinant tumor necrosis factor in metastatic breast cancer. Cancer 1991;68:1694–1695.
94 Rinehart J, Balcerzak SP, Hersh ME: Phase II trial of tumor necrosis factor in human sarcoma. Proc Am Soc Clin Oncol 1990;9:317.
95 Fiedler W, Zeller W, Peimann CJ, Weh HJ, Hossfeld DK: A phase II combination trial with recombinant human tumor necrosis factor and gamma interferon in patients with colorectal cancer. Klin Wochenschr 1991;69:261–268.
96 Sohn M, Markos-Pusztai S, Kempeni J, Richter R, Räth U, Jakse G: Experience with TNF-α and interferons in progressive advanced renal cell carcinoma (abstract). Eur Cytokine Network 1992;3:232.
97 Abbruzzese JL, Levin B, Ajani JA, Faintuch JS, Pazdur R, Saks S, Edwards C, Gutterman JU: A phase II trial of recombinant human interferon-gamma and recombinant tumor necrosis factor in patients with advanced gastrointestinal malignancies: Results of a trial terminated by excessive toxicity. J Biol Response Modif 1990;9:522–527.
98 Maeda M, Watanabe N, Yamauchi N, Tsuji Y, Niitsu Y: Successful treatment of a case of hepatocellular carcinoma with tumor necrosis factor and local hyperthermia. Gastroenterol Jpn 1991;26:774–778.
99 Raeth U, Schmid H, Karck U, Kempeni J, Schlick E, Kaufmann M: Phase II trial of recombinant human tumor necrosis factor in patients with malignant ascites from ovarian carcinomas and non-ovarian tumors with intraperitoneal spread. Proc Am Soc Clin Oncol 1991;10:187.
100 Schmid H, Kaufmann M, von Minckwitz G, Grischke EM, Bastert G, Kempeni J, Raeth U: Intraperitoneal administration of tumor necrosis factor in combination with interferon alpha or gamma in 22 patients with tumor persistence of ovarian cancer. A phase II study (abstract). Eur Cytokine Network 1992;3:246.
101 Yoshida J, Wakabayashi T, Mizuno M, Sugita K, Yoshida T, Hori S, Mori T, Sato T, Karashima A, Kurisu K, Katzuzo K, Uozumi T: Clinical effect of intra-arterial tumor necrosis factor-alpha for malignant glioma. J Neurosurg 1992;77:78–83.
102 Lienard D, Lejeune FJ, Ewalenko P: In transit metastases of malignant melanoma treated by high dose rTNF alpha in combination with interferon-gamma and melphalan in isolation perfusion. World J Surg 1992;16:234–240.
103 Lienard D, Eggermont AMM, Schraffordt Koops H, Lejeune FJ: High-dose rTNF-alpha, rIFN-gamma and melphalan in isolation perfusion produce 90% CR in melanoma in transit metastases (abstract). Eur Cytokine Network 1992;3:232.
104 Lienard D, Ewalenko P, Delmotte JJ, Renard N, Lejeune FJ: High-dose recombinant tumor necrosis factor alpha in combination with interferon gamma and melphalan in isolation perfusion of the limbs for melanoma and sarcoma. J Clin Oncol 1992;10:52–60.
105 Eggermont AMM, Lienhard D, Schraffordt Koops H, van Geel AN, Hoekstra HJ, Lejeune FJ: High-dose recombinant tumor necrosis factor alpha, gamma-interferon and melphalan in isolation perfusion of the limb in patients with irresectable soft tissue sarcoma (abstract). Eur Cytokine Network 1992;3:233.

Oncology 1994;51:154–169

*Monty H. Oppenheim*
*Michael T. Lotze*

Section of Surgical Oncology and Division of Biologic Therapy, University of Pittsburgh Medical Center, Pittsburgh Cancer Institute, Pittsburgh, Pa., USA

# Interleukin-2: Solid-Tumor Therapy

**Key Words**
Interleukin-2
Melanoma
Renal cell carcinoma
Biologic therapy
T cell growth factor
Interferon-α
Nitric oxide
Tumor necrosis factor
Lymphokine-activated killer cells
Tumor-infiltrating lymphocytes

**Abstract**
Interleukin-2 (IL-2) is a soluble factor produced by T cells that stimulates growth and activity of lymphocytes and other immune cells. First noted in murine studies, the antitumor efficacy of IL-2 has been shown to induce partial and complete regression of some tumors in human clinical trials over the past decade. Although the initial clinical success of IL-2 was in combination with lymphokine-activated killer cells, IL-2 alone has subsequently been shown to be equally efficacious. Combinations of cytokines and chemotherapies with IL-2 have been generally inconclusive and disappointing with the possible exception of interferon-α. Toxicities of IL-2 are common and often dose limiting. Symptomatic therapy has allowed patients to tolerate somewhat higher doses, but has not addressed the underlying mechanisms of these toxicities which may involve mediators such as tumor necrosis factor, interferon-γ, and nitric oxide. Clinical studies assessing these factors for their involvement in the antitumor effects of IL-2 as well as its toxicities may allow better understanding of IL-2, and perhaps lead to improved cancer therapies.

## Introduction

Interleukin-2 (IL-2) is a 15-kD glycoprotein first described by Morgan et al. [1] in 1976. While developing long-term leukemic cells for viral studies, they reported in vitro growth of T cells from normal human bone marrow using conditioned medium. Originally named T-cell growth factor (TCGF), IL-2 was first characterized as the product of mitogen-stimulated T cells that supported long-term culture of T lymphocytes. A sensitive bioassay was developed in 1978 which could detect nanogram quantities of material [2] allowing rapid progress in the study of this cytokine. In subsequent studies, IL-2 has been found to either support the growth of or to activate T cells, natural killer (NK) cells [3] (large granular lymphocytes, LGLs [4], monocytes [5], and B cells [6]). IL-2 was also found to stimulate cytotoxicity of cytotoxic T cells (CTLs) [7], NK cells [8–10], and monocytes [11]. IL-2 enhances the capacities of these cells for motility [12], and conjugate formation with other cells [13]. IL-2 also increases lung and soft-tissue lymph flow and enhances production of interferon-gamma (IFN-γ) [14], IL-1, IL-6, and tumor necrosis factor (TNF) [15–17]. Production of IL-2 is normally from T cells recognizing antigen presented in the context of MHC Class I or II molecules as well as from some activated LGLs [18]. In humans, it is encoded by a single gene [19] on chromosome 4 which produces a 133-amino-acid polypeptide with a molecular weight of 15,500.

Preclinical studies in murine models of IL-2 administration were facilitated by the cloning of the gene and sub-

Dr. Michael T. Lotze, MD, Chief
Division of Surgical Oncology, Department of Surgery
University of Pittsburgh
Terrace and Desoto Streets
Pittsburgh, PA 15261 (USA)


0030–2414/94/0512–0154
$5.00/0

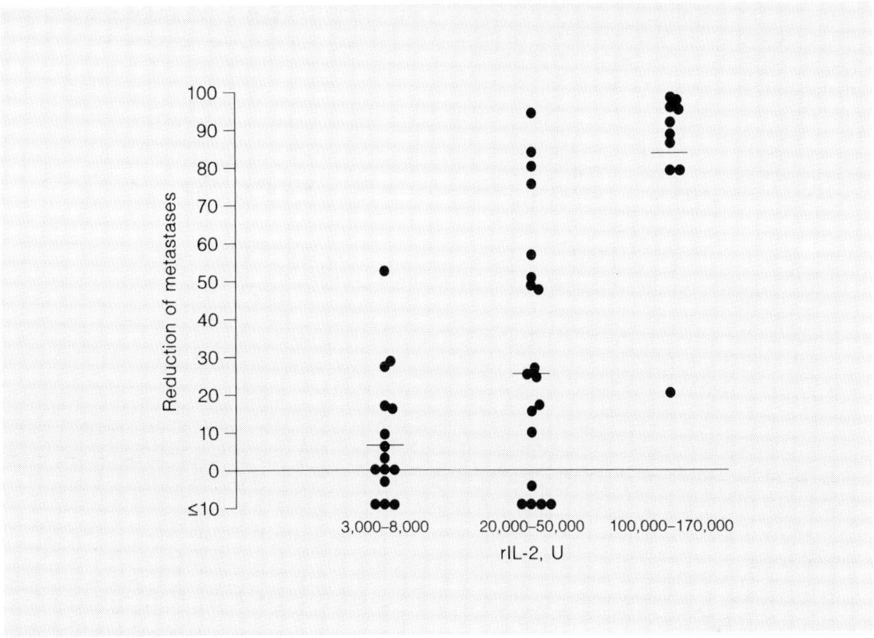


**Fig. 1.** IL-2 binding to the IL-2R complex.

sequent production of recombinant IL-2 (rIL-2) in 1983 [20, 21]. The IL-2 receptor (IL-2R) structure was also elucidated and each chain cloned [22]. Originally thought to contain only two separate proteins, an α and a β chain, IL-2R has recently been found to have a third, γ chain [23] (fig. 1). The γ chain appears to stabilize IL-2/receptor binding and probably has IL-2-binding activity itself. It is a component of high- and intermediate-affinity IL-2Rs. Recently, the IL-2Rγ gene has been localized to human chromosome Xq13 [24]. IL-2Rγ may play an important role in thymic maturation of T cells since X-linked severe combined immunodeficiency, which is characterized by absent or reduced numbers of T cells, is associated with mutations of the IL-2Rγ gene product. Cells found to express IL-2R include T cells, LGLs [8, 25], macrophages [26, 27], oligodendroglial cells [28], epidermal Langerhans' cells [29], and B cells [6, 30]. More recently some other cell lines have also been shown to express IL-2R, including squamous cell carcinoma cell lines derived from head and neck tumors, as well as some melanomas [31].

Administered intravenously in humans, IL-2 has an α half-life of 6–10 min and a β clearance phase of 30–120 min [32]. This is prolonged in intraperitoneal or subcutaneous dosing. A regimen of IL-2 dosing every 8 h has been found by pharmacokinetic studies to produce detectable levels of IL-2 throughout the study periods (>6 U/ml serum) if a dose of at least 600,000 IU (1 mg = 18 × $10^6$ IU) is used [33].

## Murine Studies of IL-2

IL-2 has been administered to animals in a variety of routes and schedules. Various approaches to dosing have been studied, including continuous infusion via intravenous catheters or with implantable osmotic pumps [34], slow release of drug by putting it into a matrix F-127 gel [35], and complexing it with polyethylene glycol (PEG) [36] to prolong its half-life. The kidney is the main site of clearance; ligation of the renal pedicle increases the half-life in mice from 2 to 84 min [33]. Radio-iodinated IL-2 has its greatest uptake in the liver and kidney [37]. By radioautography, the kidney cortex and adrenals have the greatest uptake, with homogeneous uptake in the lung, brain, and liver. IL-2 is probably also absorbed at sites of inflammation. Recently, renal allografts undergoing cellular rejection displayed enhanced retention of $^{123}$I-IL-2, presumably bound to activated T cells, when compared to nonrejecting allografts [38].

In preclinical animal models, IL-2 appears to mediate a wide range of immune effects including restoration of immune function in immunosuppressed mice [39–41], increased immunity to foreign antigens [42, 43], and increased potency of some vaccine formulations [44]. One of the first demonstrations of the systemic antitumor effects of rIL-2 was in a model of pulmonary metastases. This is summarized in figure 2 [33]. In this model C57BL/6 mice were injected intravenously with a weakly immu-

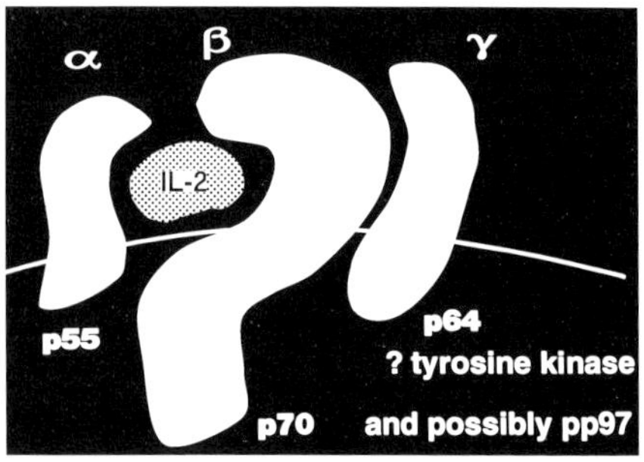


**Fig. 2.** Results of 36 consecutive experiments evaluating the ability of varying doses of rIL-2 to reduce day-3 pulmonary metastases. Each dot represents a separate experimental measurement in which mice receiving rIL-2 were compared with mice treated with Hanks' balanced salt solution alone. Therapy with varying doses of rIL-2 was initiated 3 days after intravenous injection of MCA-105 sarcoma cells. It was administered intraperitoneally approximately every 8 h for 5 days. Doses of 100,000–170,000 U of rIL-2 significantly reduced pulmonary metastases in nine of ten experiments.

nogenic sarcoma, MCA-105. At either 3 or 10 days following injection, treatment was begun with IL-2 administered for 4–5 days intraperitoneally three times a day. Micrometastatic pulmonary disease (day 3 model) only responded to the highest doses. Macroscopic disease (day 10 model) responded at lower IL-2 doses. Subsequent lung metastasis [45], experiments with different tumors, subcutaneous tumor studies [46], and liver tumor experiments [47, 48] showed similar results.

The antitumor activity of IL-2 appears to be immune mediated. Infiltrating activated lymphocytes are seen at the sites of regressing pulmonary metastases [49]. Pretreatment of animals with total-body irradiation eliminates the antitumor effects of IL-2 [50]. The lymphocyte subsets responsible for tumor rejection have been evaluated by in vivo depletion using monoclonal antibodies [51]. Different subsets are responsible for different antitumor effects: depleting ASGM-1+ cells eliminated IL-2 efficacy in treating either MCA-101 or -102 (nonimmunogenic tumors (and MCA-105 or -106 (weakly immunogenic tumors) when treatment begins on day 3 following injection of the tumor. Depletion of CD8+ cells abrogated the antitumor effects in MCA-105 or -106 10 days prior to treatment. IL-2 administration was ineffective in the treatment of day-10 nonimmunogenic tumors. Class I MHC expression appears to be required for tumor recognition. Transfecting the IL-2 treatment-insensitive B16BL6 melanoma with class I MHC genes makes it susceptible to subsequent treatment in vivo with IL-2 [52–54].

## Human Studies

The first use of IL-2 in cancer patients was reported in 1983. Partially purified IL-2 from stimulated normal lymphocytes was given to two melanoma patients [55]. rIL-2 dose escalation phase I trials began in 1984. These studies defined toxicities without apparent efficacy [17, 56]. The first patient to respond to IL-2 was simultaneously given lymphokine-activated killer (LAK) cells in 1984 and had a complete response of her metastatic melanoma persisting for over 9 years [57]. The first patient to respond to IL-2 alone was treated in 1985 [58]. Table 1 summarizes many of the recent trials of systemic IL-2 administered alone to patients with cancer. Antitumor effects were seen in these studies usually with doses of 720,000 IU/kg every 8 h, administered over 4–5 days, intravenously or intraperitoneally. Less intensive regimens appeared to be less effective. Our experience at the University of Pittsburgh utilizing a rapid-bolus IL-2 protocol (given in <1 min) has shown similar results. With 15 patients evaluable for response, objective responses have been observed in 4 of 12 patients with either metastatic renal cell carcinoma (1 of 6) or metastatic melanoma (3 of 6), one of whom had a complete response. These responses have persisted for 8, 10, 11, and 13 months to date. Responses have been observed in lung, liver, bowel, bladder, nodal, and subcutaneous-tissue metastatic sites.

## Adoptive Cellular Therapy

Adoptive cellular therapy (ACT) involves the transfer of immune cells with antitumor activity usually with concomitant IL-2 administration to the tumor-bearing host (table 2). This approach to treatment of malignancy is hampered by the difficulty of identifying cells with selective antitumor activity and producing sufficient numbers of these cells. Cells with LAK activity are lymphocytes that are capable of lysing fresh tumor without apparently harming normal cells. Derivation of this lytic activity has been observed with incubation of lymphocytes in a variety of different cytokines including IL-2, IL-4, IL-7 [116], IL-10, and IL-12. In animal models, concomitant administration of cells with LAK activity and IL-2 can cause regression of established tumors. These preclinical studies also showed that at low doses of IL-2, the combination of cells with LAK activity and IL-2 had greater antitumor effect than either component alone. Subsequent studies have questioned the value, in human trials, of the addition of LAK cells [117, 118]. Of note is our recent NCI study showing a small increase in response rate and survival with LAK administration (not statistically significant) in a randomized, prospective trial [119].

ACT has been evaluated for other cells: adherent LAK [120], macrophages [121], anti-CD3-stimulated cells [122, 123], and specific MHC-restricted CTLs [124, 125]. Tumor-infiltrating lymphocytes (TIL) are generated in vitro from most human malignancies. When derived from malignant melanoma (MM), such cells often have specific cytolytic activity against the autologous tumor. The National Biotherapy Study Group Trial, using TIL treatment for a number of different tumors, has concluded that TIL regimens, presently, are technically difficult, costly, and effective in only a minority of patients. However, using gene transfection techniques, it may be possible to alter the adoptively transferred lymphocyte functions potentiating new therapeutic options with TIL, which, unlike LAK cells, appear to traffic to tumor [126, 127].

## IL-2 plus Cytokines

Several other cytokines are being evaluated for their individual therapeutic antitumor activity and their ability to synergize with IL-2 treatment. Preclinical trials in animal models have shown enhancement of T and NK cell cytotoxicity mediated by several individual cytokines. Human protocols involving TNF-α [128], IL-4 [129], and IFN-α [130, 131], IFN-β [132], and IFN-γ [133–136] have been tried in the past few years with mixed results. The most encouraging of these combinations has been that of IL-2 with IFN-α. IFN has direct antiproliferative effects [51, 137, 138]. Synergy may occur via enhanced MHC antigen expression on tumor or effector cells exposed to IFN [139]. Although IFN alone has its greatest clinical activity in hematological malignancies, namely hairy cell leukemia and chronic myeloid leukemia, it can also mediate regression of solid tumors such as metastatic renal cell carcinoma and melanoma in 15–20% of patients [128]. It has also been approved for use in treating Kaposi's sarcoma in AIDS patients. Table 3 details the results of some of the most recent combination protocols incorporating IL-2 and IFN or other immunologic agents. These combinations share the potential for greater efficacy and/or reduced toxicity than therapy with either agent individually. To date, however, no combination therapy has yet been shown to be superior to that of high-dose IL-2 therapy alone.

## IL-2 plus Chemotherapy

Animal studies combining IL-2 with various cytotoxic agents have been cited in the available literature as having synergistic or additive antitumor reactivity. Generally, only immunogenic tumors in immunocompetent hosts seem to respond, and this is optimized if the chemotherapeutic agent is given prior to the IL-2. Postulated mechanisms for the benefit of combination therapy include the immunomodulatory properties of chemotherapies potentiating IL-2-induced immune reponse against tumor (e.g., cyclophosphamide is postulated to decrease suppressor cell activity enhancing IL-2 activation of effector cells), induction of tumor site inflammation, or tumor membrane alteration. Single chemotherapeutic agents used with IL-2 include cyclophosphamide, doxorubicin, cisplatin, dacarbazine, vinblastine, and 5-fluorouracil. Other studies have used multiagent chemotherapy and multiple immunotherapies including IL-2. Almost all of these studies are phase I or II trials. Although it is beyond the scope of this article to comprehensively review all of the literature, the results overall are best described as inconclusive and disappointing. Single-agent trials with IL-2 show the same response rates in patients with renal cell carcinoma as with combined therapies, i.e., 20–25% or less. In MM, either high-dose chemotherapy or multiagent chemotherapy with IL-2 yields about a 35% response rate, which is about what is reported for chemotherapy alone in some trials. These IL-2 response rates may be more durable. Patients with MM seem to have promising responses to IL-2 in combination with chemotherapy plus IFN-α, with response rates in the range of 45–55%, including 15–20% complete responses in some series. Duration of response has yet to be determined from these recent studies.

## Immunological and Systemic Effects/Toxicities

The efficacy of IL-2 appears to be directly related to the dose level: the higher the dose, the more likely that the patient will respond. Although this is clear in animal models, patient heterogeneity has allowed only a weak association to be made with dose of IL-2 received and antitumor response. In fact, high-dose intravenous (720,000 IU/kg, three times per day), low-dose intravenous (72,000 IU/kg, three times per day), and subcutaneous outpatient (250,000 IU/kg on days 1–5 followed by 125,000 IU/kg five days out of seven for each week for the subsequent 5 weeks) doses of IL-2 are now being compared in patients

**Table 1.** Solid-tumor response to IL-2

| Authors | Year | Dose/regimen | Diagnosis | Number of patients | CR | PR | CR + PR % |
|---|---|---|---|---|---|---|---|
| Lotze et al. [59] | 1986 | $10^4$–$3 \times 10^5$ U/kg tid, ip | melanoma | 3 | 0 | 1 | 33 |
| | | | ovarian | 1 | 0 | 0 | 0 |
| | | | colorectal | 3 | 0 | 0 | 0 |
| Rosenberg et al. [60, 61] | 1987, 1989 | $0.3 \times 10^5$–$10^5$ U/kg, q8h iv, 4–5d/w × 2w | renal cell | 54 | 4 | 8 | 22 |
| | | | melanoma | 42 | 0 | 10 | 24 |
| | | | colorectal | 12 | 0 | 0 | 0 |
| | | | non-Hodgkin's lymphoma | 11 | 0 | 0 | 0 |
| | | | breast | 3 | 0 | 0 | 0 |
| | | | other | 8 | 0 | 0 | 0 |
| Sondel et al. [62] | 1988 | $1 \times 10^6$–$3 \times 10^6$ U/m²/d ci, 4d/w × 4w | renal cell | 6 | 0 | 1 | 17 |
| | | | melanoma | 5 | 0 | 0 | 0 |
| Sosman et al. [63] | 1988 | $1 \times 10^6$–$3 \times 10^6$ U/m²/d ci or iv, 4d/w × 4w | renal cell | 17 | 0 | 3 | 18 |
| Allison et al. [64] | 1989 | $1.5 \times 10^6$–$3 \times 10^6$ U/m²/d iv, 5d, qow × 4w | melanoma | 8 | 0 | 0 | 0 |
| | | | renal cell | 2 | 0 | 0 | 0 |
| | | | colorectal | 6 | 0 | 0 | 0 |
| | | | breast | 2 | 0 | 0 | 0 |
| Creekmore et al. [65] | 1989 | 1,000–$30 \times 10^6$ U/m²/dose ci × 24h, qw | colon | 21 | 0 | 0 | 0 |
| | | | melanoma | 12 | 0 | 2 | 17 |
| Goldstein et al. [66] | 1989 | $3 \times 10^6$ U/m²d, ci 4d/w × 3w, then outpatient | renal | 9 | 0 | 0 | 0 |
| | | | melanoma | 4 | 0 | 0 | 0 |
| Ghosh et al. [67] | 1989 | MTD: $11 \times 10^6$ CU/m² intrasplenic then iv | melanoma | 31 | 0 | 4 | 13 |
| Hesh et al. [68] | 1989 | 1,000–$14 \times 10^6$ CU/m²/d iv, tiw × 8w | melanoma | 26 | 0 | 3 | 12 |
| | | | sarcoma | 12 | 0 | 0 | 0 |
| | | | colon | 7 | 0 | 0 | 0 |
| | | | head and neck | 9 | 0 | 0 | 0 |
| | | | renal cell | 4 | 0 | 0 | 0 |
| | | | other | 8 | 0 | 0 | 0 |
| Nasr et al. [69] | 1989 | $1 \times 10^6$–$3 \times 10^6$ U/m² iv, tiw × 3w | neuroblastoma | 1 | 0 | 0 | 0 |
| | | | sarcoma | 1 | 0 | 0 | 0 |
| Bajorin et al. [70] | 1990 | $3 \times 10^6$ U/m²/d, ci, iv 5d/w × 4w | renal cell | 24 | 1 | 2 | 12 |
| Bukowski et al. [71] | 1990 | $10^7$ CU/m², iv, tiw | renal cell | 44 | 1 | 4 | 11 |
| Legha et al. [72] | 1990 | $3 \times 10^6$–$4 \times 10^6$ U/m²/d, iv ci, 96h/w × 4w, q6w | melanoma | 12 | 0 | 1 | 8 |
| Lembersky et al. [73] | 1990 | $0.06 \times 10^6$–$30 \times 10^6$ IU/m²/d, ip | ovarian | 34 | | | 15 |
| | | A: ci, 24h/w, qw × 16w | | | 2 | 1 | |
| | | B: ci, 7d/w, qow × 16w | | | 1 | 1 | |
| Paciucci et al. [74] | 1990 | $20 \times 10^6$–$67.5 \times 10^6$ IU/m²/d iv, ci, 6d/2 × 4w | unspecified cancer | 41 | 0 | 13 | 32 |
| Sarna et al. [75] | 1990 | MTD: 275 U/kg qd | renal cell | 4 | 0 | 0 | 0 |
| | | | colon | 4 | 0 | 0 | 0 |
| | | | melanoma | 3 | 0 | 0 | 0 |
| | | | non-small cell lung | 1 | 0 | 0 | 0 |

**Table 1** (continued)

| Authors | Year | Dose/regimen | Diagnosis | Number of patients | CR | PR | CR + PR % |
|---|---|---|---|---|---|---|---|
| Selvaggi et al. [76] | 1990 | 1,200–120,000 IU/d × 5d × 2w perilesion and intranodal | squamous cell – head and neck | 12 | 0 | 1 | 8 |
| Stoter et al. [77] | 1990 | 5,000–1 × $10^6$ U/d, ci intrapleural × 14d | mesothelioma | 10 | | 3 | 33 |
| Atkins et al. [78] | 1991 | 0.6 × $10^6$ IU/kg/dose, q8h iv × 5d, twice in 19d | renal cell | 30 | 1 | 7 | 27 |
| Caligiuri et al. [79] | 1991 | 1.5 × $10^5$–4.5 × $10^5$ U/m$^2$/d ci × 3 months, outpatient | unspecified cancer | 13 | 0 | 0 | 0 |
| Eggermont et al. [80] | 1991 | 5,000–6 × $10^6$ IU/d, q2w intrapleural | mesothelioma | 17 | 0 | 4 | 24 |
| Israel et al. [81] | 1991 | 18 × $10^6$ U/m$^2$/d, iv, ci 5d/w × 3w | gastrointestinal | 17 | 0 | 0 | 0 |
| Matijssen et al. [82] | 1991 | 200–8,000 IU/d, qd perilymphatically × 10d | squamous cell – head and neck | 13 | 0 | 0 | 0 |
| Mertens et al. [83] | 1991 | 18 × $10^6$–36 × $10^6$ IU/m$^2$/d ci, × 5/11d, × 3 cycles | renal cell | 25 | 2 | 3 | 20 |
| Meyers et al. [84] | 1991 | MTD: 20 × $10^6$ U/m$^2$/d PEG-IL-2, iv, qw | renal cell<br>melanoma<br>prostate<br>other | 16<br>13<br>4<br>33 | 0<br>0<br>0<br>0 | 2<br>0<br>1<br>0 | 12<br>0<br>25<br>0 |
| Perez et al. [85] | 1991 | 18 × $10^6$–72 × $10^6$ IU/m$^2$/d iv, weekly | melanoma<br>renal cell | 17<br>12 | 0<br>1 | 1<br>1 | 6<br>17 |
| Poo et al. [86] | 1991 | 'NCI high-dose' q8h × 5d, twice in 15d | renal cell | 20 | 0 | 4 | 20 |
| Velotti et al. [87] | 1991 | 18,000–18 × $10^6$ IU/m$^2$/d intra-arterial, ci | transitional cell | 12 | 2 | 3 | 42 |
| Clamon et al. [88] | 1992 | 3 × $10^6$ Nutley U/m$^2$/d ci × 96h/w, ≤ 8w | small-cell lung | 24 | 5 | 1 | 50 |
| Escudier et al. [89] | 1992 | 24 × $10^6$ IU/m$^2$/d ci, 2d/2 × 5w | renal cell | 88 | 0 | 16 | 18 |
| Gore et al. [90] | 1992 | 0.03 × $10^6$–30 × $10^6$ IU/d, ci × 10d intra-arterial | squamous cell – head and neck | 12 | 0 | 2 | 17 |
| Palmer et al. [91] | 1992 | ci, iv, 20 days median | renal cell | 225 | | | 15 |
| Sleijfer et al. [92] | 1992 | 18 × $10^6$–9 × $10^6$ IU/d outpatient, sc, qd × 5d | renal cell | 26 | 2 | 4 | 23 |
| Soiffer et al. [93] | 1992 | 4.5 × $10^5$ U/m$^2$/d, ci × 8w and bolus 0.25 × $10^6$–5 × $10^6$ U/m$^2$, qw × 5w | metastatic cancer | 6 | 0 | 0 | 0 |
| Sorio et al. [94] | 1992 | 18 × $10^6$ IU/m$^2$/d, q3w × 2 ci, 5d/w × 2w | renal cell | 30 | 5 | 3 | 27 |
| Truitt et al. [95] | 1992 | 60,000–0.6 × $10^6$ IU/kg q8h × 5d | neuroblastoma solid/leukemia | 8 | 0 | 0 | 0 |

1 mg proleukin IL-2 = 3 × $10^6$ Cetus units (CU) = 18 × $10^6$ IU. CR = Complete response; PR = partial response; ti = three times per; q = every; qo = every other; d = day; w = week; ci = continuous infusion; ip = intraperitoneal; iv = intravenous; sc = subcutaneous; MTD = maximal tolerated dose; NCI = National Cancer Institute.

**Table 2.** Adoptive cellular therapy

| Authors | Year | Dose/regimen IL-2 | Dose/regimen cells | Diagnosis | Number of evaluable patients | CR | PR | CR + PR % |
|---|---|---|---|---|---|---|---|---|
| Rosenberg et al. [57] | 1985 | $0.01 \times 10^6$–$0.1 \times 10^6$ CU/kg, q8h, × 5d, × 2 cycles | LAK | melanoma | 7 | 1 | 3 | 57 |
| | | | | renal cell | 3 | 0 | 3 | 100 |
| | | | | rectal/colon | 9 | 0 | 3 | 33 |
| | | | | lung adeno | 1 | 0 | 1 | 100 |
| | | | | other | 5 | 0 | 0 | 0 |
| Rosenberg et al. [61] | 1987 | $0.1 \times 10^6$ CU/kg, q8h, × 5d, × 2 cycles | LAK | renal cell | 36 | 4 | 8 | 33 |
| | | | | melanoma | 26 | 2 | 4 | 23 |
| | | | | colorectal | 26 | 1 | 2 | 12 |
| | | | | NH lymphoma | 2 | 1 | 1 | 100 |
| | | | | other | 16 | 0 | 0 | 0 |
| West et al. [96] | 1987 | $1 \times 10^6$–$5 \times 10^6$ CU/m², ci, × 5d, ×2 cycles | LAK | melanoma | 10 | 0 | 5 | 50 |
| | | | | renal cell | 6 | 0 | 3 | 50 |
| | | | | lung | 5 | 0 | 1 | 20 |
| | | | | parotid | 2 | 0 | 1 | 50 |
| | | | | ovarian | 1 | 0 | 1 | 100 |
| | | | | lymphoma | 2 | 0 | 2 | 100 |
| | | | | other | 14 | 0 | 0 | 0 |
| Rosenberg et al. [97] | 1988 | $0.1 \times 10^6$ CU/kg, q8h, × 5d | TIL, $2 \times 10^{11}$ (max) | melanoma | 20 | 1 | 10 | 55 |
| Dutcher et al. [98] | 1989 | $0.6 \times 10^6$ IU/kg, q8h | LAK, $8.9 \times 10^{10}$ | melanoma | 32 | 1 | 5 | 19 |
| Hawkins et al. [99] | 1989 | $0.6 \times 10^6$ IU/kg, q8h | LAK | melanoma | 32 | 1 | 5 | 19 |
| | | | | colorectal | 19 | 1 | 2 | 16 |
| Koretz et al. [100] | 1989 | $3 \times 10^6$ U/m²/d, ci, 24h d1–5, 13–17, 21–24, 28–31 | LAK, 5d culture, d13–+5 | renal cell | 8 | 0 | 0 | 0 |
| | | | | melanoma | 8 | 0 | 0 | 0 |
| Margolin et al. [101] | 1989 | $8.4 \times 10^6$ IU/kg → $6 \times 10^6$ IU/kg | LAK, $7.6 \times 10^{10}$ | melanoma | 32 | 1 | 5 | 19 |
| | | | | renal cell | 35 | 2 | 3 | 16 |
| | | | | colon | 22 | 1 | 4 | 12 |
| Negrier et al. [102] | 1989 | $18 \times 10^6$ IU/m²/d | LAK | renal cell | 53 | 5 | 9 | 27 |
| Paciucci et al. [103] | 1989 | $6 \times 10^6$–$30 \times 10^6$ IU/m²/d, ci | LAK, $5.6 \times 10^9$ | melanoma | 5 | 0 | 1 | 20 |
| | | | | renal cell | 9 | 0 | 1 | 11 |
| | | | | lymphoma | 4 | 0 | 1 | 25 |
| | | | | other | 6 | 0 | 2 | 30 |
| Stahel et al. [104] | 1989 | $0.18 \times 10^6$ IU/kg/d, q8h | LAK, $5.1 \times 10^{10}$ | renal cell | 14 | 0 | 3 | 21 |
| | | | | melanoma | 7 | 0 | 1 | 14 |
| | | | | other | 5 | 0 | 0 | 0 |

with renal cell cancer at the NIH. The higher doses produce significant, occasionally even life-threatening, toxicities. Many of these toxicities appear related to a capillary leak syndrome (CLS). There is an increase in generalized vascular permeability causing egress of intravascular fluid into the interstitium of all organ systems. Although the cause of this is poorly understood, it appears from murine models that intact immune function is required and, in particular, that cells with LAK activity play a crucial role [145]. The results are evident in many organ systems.

**Table 2** (continued)

| Authors | Year | Dose/regimen IL-2 | Dose/regimen cells | Diagnosis | Number of evaluable patients | CR | PR | CR + PR % |
|---|---|---|---|---|---|---|---|---|
| Thompson et al. [105] | 1989 | 6 × $10^6$ IU/m$^2$/d, q8h | LAK, 3.4 × $10^{10}$ | melanoma | 4 | 0 | 0 | 0 |
| | | | | renal cell | 3 | 0 | 0 | 0 |
| | | | | colorectal | 4 | 0 | 0 | 0 |
| | | 18 × $10^6$ IU/m$^2$/d, ci | LAK, 4.3 × $10^{10}$ | melanoma | 4 | 0 | 0 | 0 |
| | | | | renal cell | 8 | 1 | 0 | 13 |
| Hanson et al. [107] | 1990 | 3 × $10^6$–6 × $10^6$ U/m$^2$/d, ci, 5d → 3 × $10^6$–4.5 × $10^6$ U/m$^2$/d, iv, 5d | LAK, 5d culture | renal cell + melanoma + others | 17 | 0 | 0 | 0 |
| Parkinson et al. [108] | 1990 | 0.6 × $10^6$ IU/m$^2$ × 3d bolus → 18 × $10^6$ IU/m$^2$ × 6d, ci | LAK | renal cell | 47 | 2 | 2 | 9 |
| Steiss et al. [109] | 1990 | 0.1 × $10^6$ U/kg, iv, q8h, × 3d → 25,000 U/kg, q8h, × 5d, ip | LAK, 7d culture, ip | ovarian | 10 | 0 | 2 | 20 |
| | | | | colorectal | 12 | 0 | 5 | 42 |
| | | | | others | 2 | 0 | 0 | 0 |
| Usui et al. [110] | 1990 | | LAK | renal cell | 9 | 0 | 1 | 11 |
| Dillman et al. [111] | 1991 | 18 × $10^6$ IU/m$^2$/d, ci, × 96h | TIL, $10^{11}$ | melanoma | 21 | 1 | 4 | 24 |
| Dutcher et al. [106] | 1991 | ci, iv, 0.18 × $10^6$ IU/m$^2$/d | LAK, ci, iv | melanoma | 33 | 0 | 1 | 3 |
| Han [112] | 1991 | 0.2 × $10^6$–0.3 × $10^6$ IU/d d1,2,8,9,10 iv | LAK (1–2 × $10^9$), via hepatic artery or hLAK (0.5 × $10^9$–1 × $10^9$), iv | liver, primary | 5 | 0 | 3 | 60 |
| | | | | liver, metastatic | 5 | 2 | 1 | 60 |
| Hayes et al. [113] | 1991 | Intracavitary, tiw via Ommaya reservoir | | glioma | 9 | 0 | 2 | 22 |
| Foon et al. [114] | 1992 | 6 × $10^6$ IU/m$^2$/d, ci | LAK, ex vivo, cultured with phenylalanine methyl | renal cell | 23 | 2 | 4 | 26 |
| Weiss et al. [115] | 1992 | A: bolus, tid | LAK, 3–4d culture | renal cell | 46 | 3 | 6 | 20 |
| | | B: ci, × 24h | LAK, 3–4d culture | renal cell | 48 | 2 | 5 | 15 |

1 mg proleukin IL-2 = 3 × $10^6$ Cetus units (CU) = 18 × $10^6$ IU. CR = Complete response; PR = partial response; ti = three times per; q = every; h = hour; d = day; w = week; ci = continuous infusion; iv = intravenous; ip = intraperitoneal; max = maximum; LAK = (autologous) lymphokine-activated killer cells; hLAK = homologous LAK; TIL = tumor-infiltrating lymphocytes; NH = non-Hodgkin's.

Generally, there is a variable weight gain of up to 10–20% of original body weight within 3 to 4 days of treatment. This is manifested as peripheral edema, pleural effusions, and ascites. CLS results in hypotension often requiring pressor support and fluids, oliguria, azotemia, respiratory failure occasionally requiring intubation, and neurological abnormalities including agitation, disorientation, obtundation, and, occasionally, coma.

Other specific toxicities include cardiovascular toxicities with supraventricular and ventricular arrhythmias,

**Table 3.** Solid-tumor response to IL-2 used with other immunologic agents

| Authors | Year | Dose/regimen: IL-2 | Dose/regimen: other immunologic agent | Diagnosis | Number of evaluable patients | CR | PR | CR + PR % |
|---|---|---|---|---|---|---|---|---|
| Rosenberg et al. [130] | 1989 | $1 \times 10^6$–$4.5 \times 10^6$ U/m$^2$/d iv, q8h, × 5d | *IFN-α* $3 \times 10^6$–$6 \times 10^6$ U/m$^2$/d, iv, q8h, × 5d | melanoma<br>renal cell<br>colorectal<br>other | 39<br>35<br>9<br>8 | 3<br>4<br>0<br>0 | 10<br>7<br>1<br>0 | 33<br>31<br>11<br>0 |
| Atzpodien et al. [140] | 1990 | $9 \times 10^6$ IU/m$^2$ q12h × 2d then $1.8 \times 10^6$ IU/m$^2$ 5d/w × 6w, all sc | *IFN-α2b* sc, $5 \times 10^6$ U/m$^2$, 3d/w × 6w | renal cell | 14 | 2 | 3 | 36 |
| Bajorin et al. [141] | 1990 | $1 \times 10^6$ U/m$^2$/dose, iv in 6h, × 5d, × 2 cycles | *MAb R24* 1–12 mg/m$^2$/d | melanoma | 20 | 0 | 1 | 5 |
| Krigel et al. [132] | 1990 out-pt | $30 \times 10^6$ IU/m$^2$/d, iv, tiw | *IFN-β* iv, $6 \times 10^6$ U/m$^2$/d | renal cell | 22 | 1 | 5 | 27 |
| Redman et al. [135] | 1990 | MTD = $1 \times 10^6$ IU/m$^2$ ci, 5d/2w, × 3 | *IFN-γ* MTD = $8 \times 10^6$ U/m$^2$/d, im, 5d/2w, × 3 | renal cell<br>NH lymphoma<br>melanoma<br>other | 6<br>4<br>1<br>15 | 0<br>0<br>0<br>0 | 0<br>1<br>0<br>0 | 0<br>25<br>0<br>0 |
| Yang et al. [128] | 1990 | $6 \times 10^6$ IU/m2h2/d ci, × 5d | *TNF-α* im, 25–100 μg/m$^2$/d, × 5d | non-small cell lung | 12 | 0 | 1 | 8 |
| Atkins et al. [78] | 1991 | 0.8 mg/m$^2$/dose iv, q8h, d1–5, 15–19 | *IFN-α2b* $3 \times 10^6$ U/m$^2$/dose iv, q8h, d1–5, 15–19 | renal cell | 28 | 0 | 3 | 11 |
| Atzpodien and Kirchner [142] | 1991 out-pt | $14.4 \times 10^6$–$18 \times 10^6$ U/m$^2$ × 2d, $3.6 \times 10^6$–$4.8 \times 10^6$ U/m$^2$ × 3d qw, × 6w | *IFN-α2b* $3 \times 10^6$–$6 \times 10^6$ U/m$^2$ 2–3/2, × 6w | renal cell<br>melanoma<br>other | 32<br>12<br>10 | 4<br>0<br>0 | 6<br>1<br>0 | 31<br>8<br>0 |

myocarditis, ischemia, and even myocardial infarction in 1–4% of patients [146]. Gastrointestinal toxicities, although not usually dose limiting, are among the most common and most trying for these patients. These include nausea, vomiting, and diarrhea occurring in most patients. TNF-α, which is known to be released into the circulation of IL-2-treated patients, may be involved in these as well as in IL-2-induced anorexia and fevers [147]. Peptic ulcer disease and colonic infarctions and perforations have been documented. Elevations in liver function tests are almost always seen and reversible cholestasis is common [148].

Other toxicities occasionally seen with IL-2 therapy include hypothyroidism [149], macular erythema with pruritis followed by desquamation [150], anemia requiring transfusion in as many as 50% of patients [101] and thrombocytopenia below 20,000/μl in 20% of patients [60], fevers, chills, and an increased incidence of bacterial infection in 10 to 30% of patients [6, 29].

It is important to note that most of these toxicities will begin to reverse within 24 h of cessation of IL-2 therapy with complete resolution usually within a few days to a week. Nonetheless, many efforts have been made to reduce the dose-limiting toxicities and improve the tolerability of IL-2 therapy. These efforts include careful patient selection and use of concomitant medications designed to ameliorate these side effects.

**Table 3** (continued)

| Authors | Year | Dose/regimen IL-2 | other immunologic agent | Diagnosis | Number of evaluable patients | CR | PR | CR + PR % |
|---|---|---|---|---|---|---|---|---|
| Figlin et al. [131] | 1992 | $2 \times 10^6$ IU/m²/d ci, × 4d | *IFN-α2a* $2 \times 10^6$ U/m²/d | renal cell | 30 | 3[1] | 9 | 30 |
| Fiorentino et al. [143] | 1992 out-pt | $0.24 \times 10^6$–$2.4 \times 10^6$ IU/m²/d, sc, × 5d on second w | *IFN-α2b* $3 \times 10^6$ U/m²/d, × 5d | renal cell | 12 | 0 | 0 | 0 |
| Margolin et al. [133] | 1992 out-pt | $6 \times 10^6$–$42 \times 10^6$ IU/m²/d | *IFN-γ* $1 \times 10^6$–$4 \times 10^6$ U/m²/d | renal cell | 6 | 0 | 0 | 0 |
| | | | | melanoma | 6 | 0 | 1 | 17 |
| | | | | colorectal | 6 | 0 | 0 | 0 |
| | | | | lung | 2 | 0 | 1 | 50 |
| | | | | other | 6 | 0 | 0 | 0 |
| Taylor et al. [134] | 1992 out-pt | $12 \times 10^6$–$24 \times 10^6$ IU/m²/d, iv, d8–12 | *IFN-γ* im, $2 \times 10^6$–$4 \times 10^6$ U/m²/d | renal cell | 11 | 1 | 0 | 9 |
| | | | | melanoma | 7 | 0 | 1 | 14 |
| | | | | GI | 5 | 0 | 0 | 0 |
| | | | | other | 14 | 0 | 0 | 0 |
| Viens et al. [136] | 1992 | $8 \times 10^6$ IU/m²/dose, q8h × 5d, q12h × 5d | *IFN-γ* $1 \times 10^6$–$10 \times 10^6$ U/m²/d qod, × 3–5/cycle | melanoma | 11 | 1 | 1 | 18 |
| | | | | renal cell | 5 | 0 | 1 | 20 |
| | | | | NH lymphoma | 2 | 0 | 1 | 50 |
| | | | | other | 9 | 0 | 0 | 0 |
| Ziegler et al. [144] | 1992 | $2 \times 10^6$–$4.5 \times 10^6$ U/m²/d, sc, × 4d, × 3w | *MAb L6* 200 mg/m²/d, d1–7 | breast | 5 | 0 | 0 | 0 |
| | | | | colorectum | 5 | 0 | 1 | 20 |
| | | | | lung | 5 | 0 | 0 | 0 |

1 mg proleukin IL-2 = $3 \times 10^6$ Cetus units (CU) = $18 \times 10^6$ IU. CR = Complete response; PR = partial response; out-pt = outpatient; ti = three times per; q = every; qo = every other; h = hour; d = day; w = week; ci = continuous infusion; iv = intravenous; sc = subcutaneous; im = intramuscular; MTD = maximal tolerated dose; MAb = monoclonal antibody; NH = non-Hodgkin's; GI = gastrointestinal.

1 Two pathological and one surgical complete response.

## Care of Patients: Selection and Concomitant Medications

Thorough prescreening evaluations of IL-2 candidates are necessary to reduce the likelihood of serious complications. Patients with CNS metastases or other neurological disease, or significant cardiac, pulmonary, or renal disease should be excluded from therapy.

As specific toxicities were identified during the early years of IL-2 therapy experience, concomitant medications have been added to control them. Acetoaminophen and indomethacin were given to ameliorate fevers, meperidine for chills, $H_2$-blockers for peptic ulcer prophylaxis, vasopressors for hypotension, and so on: treating symptomatic toxicities as they manifested themselves with what has become a long list of medications. This has allowed increases in the number of doses of IL-2, but major toxicities are almost always observed when the patient treatment strategy is to treat to the dose-limiting toxicity.

Many investigators believe that further toxicity reduction will increase efficacy by allowing higher doses of IL-2 to be administered. Various mediators of IL-2 toxicities have been suggested including TNF-α [151], IL-1 [152], and nitric oxide [153, 154]. Neutralizing antibodies and various inhibitors of these products have been and are being evaluated in animal and human studies [155, 156]. Of major concern is the possibility that these toxicity

**Table 4.** IL-2-responsive tumors

| |
|---|
| Moderately responsive |
| Melanoma |
| Renal cell carcinoma |
| Lymphoma |
| Occasionally responsive |
| Colorectal carcinoma |
| Small cell lung carcinoma |
| Hepatoma |
| Cutaneous T cell lymphoma |
| Thymoma |
| Rarely responsive |
| Breast cancer |

mediators are equally responsible for IL-2 efficacy [157]. Approaches to reduce these factors as well as utilizing treatments directed at reducing symptomatic toxicities must be evaluated for their immune function as well as their toxicity-reducing activity.

## Conclusions and Future Directions

The clinical use of IL-2 was begun enthusiastically, following impressive preclinical results showing significant immunomodulatory effects in combination with the adoptive transfer of cells as well as antitumor activity in animals. Single-agent use of IL-2 in human trials has shown significant, but low rates of antitumor responses, mostly in melanoma and renal cell carcinoma (table 4). Since its inception in broad clinical rials in 1984, multiple attempts to improve efficacy and reduce toxicity have been carried out. Few real advances other than insights related to holding therapy for certain prodromal toxicities have been observed. ACT, although associated with the first IL-2 responses, has yet to be shown to be an improvement over IL-2 therapy alone [70, 102, 111]. Similarly, combinations of IL-2 with chemotherapeutic agents have been disappointing. So far, IFN alone appears to minimally improve response rates of specific cancers to IL-2 therapy. Other methods of improving response rates have been based on the concept that higher doses of IL-2 will improve efficacy. This has led to trials of toxicity-reducing drugs administered concomitantly with IL-2 therapy, such as pentoxifylline, a xanthene derivative which reduces TNF [158] production and *n*-monomethyl-*l*-arginine [159] or aminoguanidine [160] which reduce nitric oxide synthesis through inhibition of nitric oxide synthase.

Prospects for improvement of IL-2-based therapy include several exciting possibilities. The potential to genetically alter cells used for ACT with cytotoxic or immunomodulatory genes raises the possibility of specifically targeting tumors with cells which can produce high local levels of various cytokines including IL-2 [161], IL-4 [162], G-CSF, TNF, IL-10 [163], or IL-12 [164]. This novel approach is being studied preclinically using not only T helper cells, but tumor cells alone or admixed with fibroblasts as part of tumor vaccines.

Understanding the mechanisms underlying the antitumor effects of IL-2 as well as its toxicities may allow a more directed therapy. Separating out the mediators of these responses and stimulating or inhibiting them, respectively, may allow more specific delivery of higher doses of IL-2 producing a more significant number of durable responses, which is the common goal of all these studies.

## References


1 Morgan DA, Ruscetti FW, Gallo RG: Selective in vitro growth of T-lymphocytes from normal bone marrows. Science 1976;193:1007–1008.
2 Gillis S, Ferm MM, Ou W, Smith KA: T cell growth factor: Parameters of production and a quantitative microassay for activity. J Immunol 1978;120:2027–2031.
3 Henney CS, Kuribayashi K, Kern DE, Gillis S: Interleukin-2 augments natural killer cell activity. Nature 1981;291:335.
4 Grimm EA, Robb RJ, Roth JA, Neckers LM, Lachmann LB, Wilson DJ, Rosenberg SA: Lymphokine activated killer cell phenomenon. III. Evidence that IL-2 is sufficient for direct activation of peripheral blood lymphoctes into lymphokine-activated killer cells. J Exp Med 1983;158:1356–1361.
5 Herrmann F, Cannistra SA, Lindemann A, Blohm D, Rambaldi A, Mertelsmann RH, Griffin JD: Functional consequences of monocyte IL-2 receptor expression. Induction of IL-1 beta secretion by IFN-gamma and IL-2. J Immunol 1989;142:139.
6 Zubler RH, Lowenthal JW, Erard F, Hashimoto N, Devos R, MacDonald HR: Activated B cells express receptors for, and proliferate in response to, pure interleukin-2. J Exp Med 1984;160:1170–1183.
7 Erard F, Corthesy P, Nabholz M, Lowenthal JW, Zaech P, Plaetinck G, MacDonald HR: Interleukin-2 is both necessary and sufficient for the growth and differentiation of lectin-stimulated cytolytic T lymphocyte precursors. J Immunol 1985;134:1644.

8 Lotze MT, Grimm EA, Mazumder A, Strausser JL, Rosenberg SA: Lysis of fresh and cultured autologous tumor by human lymphocytes cultured in T-cell growth factor. Cancer Res 1981; 41:4420–4425.

9 Grimm EA, Maxumder A, Zhang HZ, Rosenberg SA: Lymphokine-activated killer cell phenomenon. Lysis of natural killer-resistant fresh solid tumor cells by interleukin-2 activated autologous human peripheral blood lymphocytes. J Exp Med 1982;155:1823.

10 Jablons D, Bolton E, Mertins S, Rubin M, Pizzo P, Rosenberg SA, Lotze MT: IL-2 based immunotherapy alters circulating neutrophil Fc receptor expression and chemotaxis. J Immunol 1990;144:3630.

11 Malkovsky M, Loveland B, North M, Asherson GL, Gao L, Ward P, Fiers W: Recombinant interleukin-2 directly augments the cytotoxicity of human monocytes. Nature 1987;325:262.

12 Robbins RA, Klassen L, Rasmussen J, Clayton ME, Russ WD: Interleukin-2-induced chemotaxis of human T-lymphocytes. J Lab Clin Med 1986;108:340–345.

13 Roberts K, Lotze MT: Interleukin-2 promotes conjugate formation by purified LAK precursors and T lymphocytes: Evaluation of conjugates using flow cytometric techniques. J Biol Response Modif 1988;7:249–266.

14 Reem GH, Yeh NH: Interleukin-2 regulates expression of its receptor and synthesis of gamma interferon by human T lymphocytes. Science 1984;225:429–430.

15 Balkwill FR, Burke F: The cytokine network. Immunol Today 1989;10:299.

16 Ortaldo JR: Cytokine production by CD3– large granular lymphocyes; in Reynolds CW, Wiltrout RH (eds): Functions of the Natural Immune System. New York, Plenum, 1989, p 299.

17 Lotze MT, Matory YL, Ettinghausen SE, Rayner AA, Sharrow SO, Seipp CA, Custer MC, Rosenberg SA: In vivo administration of purified human interleukin-2. II. Half-life, immunologic effects, and expansion of peripheral lymphoid cells in vivo with recombinant IL-2. J Immunol 1985;135:2865–2875.

18 Lotze MT: Interleukin-2: Basic principles. In DeVita VT Jr, Hellman S, Rosenberg SA (eds): Biologic Therapy of Cancer. Philadelphia, Lippincott, 1991, pp 123–141.

19 Shows T, Eddy R, Haley L, Byers M, Henry M, Fujita T, Matsui H, Taniguchi T: Interleukin-2 (IL-2) is assigned to human chromosome 4. Somat Cell Mol Genet 1984;10:315–318.

20 Taniguchi T, Matsui H, Fujita T, Takaoka C, Kashima N, Yoshimoto R, Hamuro J: Structure and expression of a cloned cDNA for human interleukin-2. Nature 1983;302:305–309.

21 Rosenberg SA, Grimm EA, McGrogan M, Doyle M, Kawasaki E, Koths K, Mark DF: Biological activity of recombinant human interleukin-2 produced in *E. coli.* Science 1984;223: 1412–1414.

22 Hatakeyama M, Tsudo M, Minamoto S, Kono T, Doi T, Miyata T, Miyasaka M, Taniguchi T: Interleukin-2 receptor beta chain gene: Generation of three receptor forms by cloned human alpha and beta chain cDNAs. Science 1989; 244:551–556.

23 Sugamura K, Asao H, Suzuki J, Takeshita T: Identification of a third component, gamma chain (p 64), of interleukin-2 receptor. Serono Symp Publ Raven Press 1990;68:145.

24 Noguchi M, Huafang Y, Rosenblatt HM, Filipovich AH, Adelstein S, Modi WS, McBride OW, Leonard WJ: Interleukin-2 receptor γ chain mutation results in X-linked severe combined immunodeficiency in humans. Cell 1993;73:147–157.

25 Rosenstein M, Yron I, Kaufmann Y, Rosenberg SA: Lymphokine activated killer cells: Lysis of fresh syngeneic NK-resistant murine tumor cells by lymphocytes cultured in interleukin-2. Cancer Res 1984;44:1946–1953.

26 Holter W, Grunow R, Stockinger H, Knapp W: Recombinant interferon-gamma induces interleukin-2 receptors on human peripheral blood monocytes. J Immunol 1986;136:2171–2175.

27 Lotze MT, Custer MC, Sharrow SO, Rubin LA, Nelson DL, Rosenberg SA: In vivo administration of purified human interleukin-2 to patients with cancer: Development of interleukin-2 receptor positive cells and circulating soluble interleukin-2 receptors following interleukin-2 administration. Cancer Res 1987;47:2188–2195.

28 Benveniste EN, Merrill JE: Stimulation of oligodendroglial proliferation and maturation by interleukin-2. Nature 1986;321:610–613.

29 Steiner G, Tschachler E, Tani M, Malek TR, Shevach EM, Holter W, Knopp W, Wolff K, Stingl G: Interleukin-2 receptors on cultured murine epidermal Langerhans cells. J Immunol 1986;137:155–159.

30 Boyd AW, Fisher DC, Fox DA, Schlossman SF, Nadler LM: Structural and functional characterization of IL-2 receptors on activated human B cells. J Immunol 1985;134:2387–2392.

31 Weidemann E, Sacchi M, Plaisance S, Heo DS, Yasumura S, Lin WC, Johnson JT, Herberman RB, Azzarone B, Whiteside TL: Receptors for interleukin 2 on human squamous cell carcinoma cell lines and tumor in situ. Cancer Res 1992;52:5963.

32 Lotze MT, Frana LW, Sharrow SO, Robb RJ, Rosenberg SA: In vivo administration of purified human interleukin-2. I. Half-life and immunologic effects of the Jurkat cell line-derived interleukin-2. J Immunol 1985;134:157–166.

33 Müle J, Rosenberg SA: Interleukin-2: Preclinical trials; in De Vita VT Jr, Hellman S, Rosenberg SA (eds): Biologic Therapy of Cancer. Philadelphia, Lippincott, 1991, pp 142–158.

34 Nishimura T, Uchiyama Y, Yagi H, Hashimoto Y: Administration of slowly released recombinant interleukin-2: Augmentation of the efficacy of adoptive immunotherapy with lymphokine-activated killer (LAK) cells. J Immunol Methods 1986;91:21–27.

35 Morikawa K, Okada F, Hosokawa M, Kobayashi H: Enhancement of therapeutic effects of recombinant interleukin-2 on a transplantable rat fibrosarcoma by the use of a sustained release vehicle, pluronic gel. Cancer Res 1987; 47:37–41.

36 Katre NV, Knauf MJ, Laird WJ: Chemical modification of recombinant interleukin-2 by polyethylene glycol increases its potency in the murine Meth A sarcoma model. Proc Natl Acad Sci USA 1987;84:1487–1491.

37 Gennuso R, Spigelman MK, Vallabhajosula S, Moore F, Zappulla RA, Nieves J, Strauchen JA, Paciucci PA, Malis LI, Goldsmith SJ: Systemic biodistribution of radio-iodinated interleukin-2 in the rat. J Biol Response Modif 1989;8:375–384.

38 Abbs IC, Pratt JR, Dallman MJ, Sacks SH: Analysis of activated T cell infiltrates in rat renal allografts by gamma camera imaging after injection of $^{123}$iodine interleukin 2. Transplant Immunol 1993;1:45–51.

39 Wagner H, Hardt C, Heeg K, Rollinghoff M, Pfizenmaier K: T-cell derived helper factor allows in vivo induction of cytotoxic T cells in nu/nu mice. Nature 1980;284:278–280.

40 Thoman ML, Weigle WO: Reconstitution of in vivo cell-mediated lympholysis responses in aged mice with interleukin-2. J Immunol 1985; 134:949–952.

41 Merluzzi VJ, Kenney RE, Schmid FA, Choi YS, Faanes RB: Recovery of the in vivo cytotoxic T-cell response in cyclophosphamide treated mice by injection of mixed-lymphocyte-culture supernatants. Cancer Res 1981;41: 3663–3665.

42 Rosenberg SA, Spiess PJ, Schwarz SL: In vivo administration of interleukin-2 enhances specific alloimmune responses. Transplantation 1983;35:631–634.

43 Conlon M, Hefeneider PJ, Gillis S: The effects of interleukin-2 (IL-2) on primary in vivo immune responses. Cell Immunol 1982;70:407–413.

44 Nunberg JH, Doyle MV, York SM, York CJ: Interleukin-2 acts as an adjuvant to increase the potency of inactivated rabies virus vaccine. Proc Natl Acad Sci USA 1989;86:4240–4243.

45 Papa MZ, Müle JJ, Rosenberg SA: The antitumor efficacy of lymphokine-activated killer cells and recombinant interleukin-2 in vivo: Successful immunotherapy of established pulmonary metastases from weakly- and non-immunogenic murine tumors of three distinct histologic types. Cancer Res 1986;46:4973–4978.

46 Bubenik J, Indrova M, Toulcova A: Immunotherapy of murine sarcomas with interleukin-2. I. Local administration of human recombinant IL-2 preparations. Folia Biol (Praha) 1986;32: 384–391.

47 Lafreniere R, Rosenberg SA: Successful immunotherapy of murine experimental hepatic metastases with lymphokine-activated killer cells and recombinant interleukin-2. Cancer Res 1985;45:3735–3741.

48 Lafreniere R, Rosenberg SA: Adoptive immunotherapy of murine hepatic metastases with lymphokine-activated killer (LAK) cells and recombinant interleukin-2 (rIL-2) can mediate the regression of both immunogenic and nonimmunogenic sarcomas and an adenocarcinoma. J Immunol 1985;135:4273–4280.
49 Rosenberg SA, Müle JJ, Spiess PJ, Reichert CM, Schwartz SL: Regression of established pulmonary metastases and subcutaneous tumor mediated by the systemic administration of high-dose recombinant interleukin-2. J Exp Med 1985;161:1169–1188.
50 Rosenberg SA, Müle JJ: Immunotherapy of cancer with lymphokine-activated killer cells and recombinant interleukin-2. Surgery 1985; 98:437–443.
51 Müle JJ, Yang JC, Lafreniere RL, Shu SY, Rosenberg SA: Identification of cellular mechanisms operational in vivo during the regression of established pulmonary metastases by the systemic administration of high-dose recombinant interleukin-2. J Immunol 1987;139: 285–294.
52 Tanaka K, Hayashi H, Hamada C, Khoury G, Jay G: Expression of major histocompatibility complex class I antigens as a strategy for the potentiation of immune recognition of tumor cells. Proc Natl Acad Sci USA 1986;83:8723–8727.
53 Hui K, Grosveld F, Festenstein H: Rejection of transplantable AKR leukemia cells following MHC DNA-mediated cell transformation. Nature 1985;311:750–753.
54 Tanaka K, Isselbacher KJ, Khoury G, Jay G: Reversal of oncogenesis by the expression of a major histocompatibility complex class I gene. Science 1985;228:26–30.
55 Lotze MT, Robb RJ, Sharrow SO, Frana LW, Rosenberg SA: Systemic administration of interleukin-2 in man. J Biol Response Modif 1984;3:475–482.
56 Lotze MT, Matory YL, Rayner AA, Ettinghausen SE, Vetto JT, Seipp CA, Rosenberg SA: Clinical effects and toxicity of interleukin-2 in patients with cancer. Cancer 1986;58:2764–2772.
57 Rosenberg SA, Lotze MT, Muul LM, Leitman S, Chang AE, Ettinghausen SE, Matory YL, Skibber JM, Shiloni E, Vetto JT: Observations on the systemic administration of autologous lymphokine-activated killer cells and recombinant interleukin-2 to patients with metastatic cancer. N Engl J Med 1985;313:1485–1492.
58 Lotze MT, Chang AE, Seipp CA, Simpson C, Vetto JT, Rosenberg SA: High-dose recombinant interleukin-2 in the treatment of patients with disseminated cancer. JAMA 1986;256: 3117–3124.
59 Lotze MT, Custer MC, Rosenberg SA: Intraperitoneal administration of IL-2 in patients with cancer. Arch Surg 1986;121:1373.
60 Rosenberg SA, Lotze M, Yang JC, Aebersold PM, Linehan WM, Seipp CA, White DE: Experience with the use of high dose interleukin-2 in the treatment of 652 cancer patients. Ann Surg 1989;210:474.
61 Rosenberg SA, Lotze MT, Muul LM, Chang AE, Avis FP, Leitman S, Linehan WM, Robertson CN, Lee RE, Rubin JT: A progress report on the treatment of 157 patients with advanced cancer using lymphokine-activated killer cells and interleukin-2 or high dose interleukin-2 alone. N Engl J Med 1987;316:889–897.
62 Sondel PM, Kohler PC, Hank JA, Moore KH, Rosenthal NS, Sosman JA, Bechhofer R, Storer B: Clinical and immunological effects of recombinant interleukin-2 given by repetitive weekly cycles to patients with cancer. Cancer Res 1988;48:2561–2567.
63 Sosman JA, Kohler PC, Hank JA, Moore KH, Bechhofer R, Storer B, Sondel PM: Repetitive weekly cycles of recombinant human interleukin-2: Responses of renal carcinoma with acceptable toxicity. J Natl Cancer Inst 1988;80: 60–63.
64 Allison MAK, Jones SE, McGuffey P: Phase II trial of outpatient interleukin-2 in malignant lymphoma, chronic lymphocytic leukemia, and selected solid tumors. J Clin Oncol 1989;7:75.
65 Creekmore SP, Harris JE, Ellis TM, Braun DP, Cohen II, Bhoopalam N, Jassak PF, Cahill MA, Canzoneri CL, Fisher RI: A phase I clinical trial of recombinant interleukin-2 by periodic 24-hour intravenous infusions. J Clin Oncol 1989;7:276.
66 Goldstein D, Sosman JA, Hank JA, Weil-Hillman G, Moore KH, Borchert A, Bechhofer R, Storer B, Kohler PC, Levitt D: Repetitive weekly cycles of interleukin-2: Effect of outpatient treatment with a lower dose of interleukin-2 on non-major histocompatibility complex-restricted killer activity. Cancer Res 1989; 49:6832.
67 Ghosh AK, Dazzi H, Thatcher N, Moore M: Lack of correlation between peripheral blood lymphokine activated killer cell function and clinical response in patients with advanced malignant melanoma receiving recombinant interleukin-2. Int J Cancer 1989;43:410.
68 Hersh EM, Murray H, Hong WK, Rosenblum MG, Reuben JM, Weilbaecher R, Sarwal AN, Bradley EC, Konrad M, Arnett FC: Phase I study of cancer therapy with recombinant interleukin-2 administered by intravenous bolus injection. Biotherapy 1989;1:215.
69 Nars S, McKolanus J, Pais R, Findley H, Hnath R, Waldrep K, Ragab AH: A phase I study of interleukin-2 in children with cancer and evaluation of clinical and immunologic status during therapy. A Pediatric Oncology Group study. Cancer 1989;64:783.
70 Bajorin DF, Sell KW, Richards JM, Walther PJ, O'Connell M, Motzer R, Vogelzang NJ, Zeffren J, Levitt D: A randomized trial of interleukin-2 plus lymphokine activated killer cells versus interleukin-2 alone in renal cell carcinoma. Proc Annu Meet Am Assoc Cancer Res 1990;31:A1106.
71 Bukowski RM, Goodman P, Crawford ED, Sergi JS, Redman BG, Whitehead RP: Phase II trial of high-dose intermittent interleukin-2 in metastastic renal cell carcinoma: A Southwest Oncology Group study. J Natl Cancer Inst 1990;82:143.
72 Legha S, Gianan M, Plager C, Papadopoulos N, Salem P, Benjamin RS: Phase I-II study of IL-2 used as a continuous infusion in patients with metastatic melanoma (abstract). Proc Annu Meet Am Assoc Cancer Res 1990;31:A1047.
73 Lembersky B, Baldisseri M, Seski J, Kunschner A, Hammond R, Zook-Enk D, Vaccarello L, Bhiteside T, Herberman R, Kirkwood J: Phase IB study of intraperitoneal (IP) interleukin-2 (IL-2) for refractory ovarian cancer (OC) (abstract). Proc Annu Meet Am Assoc Cancer Res 1990;31:A1643.
74 Paciucci PA, Ryder JS, Holland JF: Correlation between clinical activity of IL-2 and antitumor effects in vitro during the first week of therapy (abstract). Proc Annu Meet Am Soc Clin Oncol 1990;9:A777.
75 Sarna G, Collins J, Figlin R, Robertson P, Altrock B, Abels R: A pilot study of intralymphatic interleukin-2. II. Clinical and biological effects. J Biol Response Modif 1990;9:81.
76 Selvaggi KJ, Vlock DR, Johnson JT, Snyderman CH, Rubin J, Kirkwood J, Haselow R, Letessier E, Whiteside T, Prescott K: Phase IB trial of peritumoral and intranodal injections of IL-2 in patients with advanced squamous cell caricnoma of the head and neck (SCCHN): Preliminary results (abstract). Proc Annu Meet Am Soc Clin Oncol 1990;9:A691.
77 Stoter G, Goey SH, Slingerland R, Bolhuis RL, Eggermont AM: Intrapleural interleukin-2 (IL-2) in malignant pleural mesothelioma: A phase I–II study (abstract). Proc Annu Meet Am Assoc Cancer Res 1990;31:A1630.
78 Atkins MB, Sparano J, Fisher RI, Weiss GR, Margolin KA, Aronson FR, Sznol M: Randomized phase II trial of high-dose IL-2 either alone or in combination with interferon alpha 2B (dfn) in advanced renal cell carcinoma (rcca) (abstract). Proc Annu Meet Am Soc Clon Oncol 1991;10:A526.
79 Caligiuri M, Canning C, Klumpp T, Soiffer R, Seiden M, Ish C, Buchanan L, Perillo Smith K, Ritz J: Phase I study of a 3-month low-dose continuous infusion of interleukin-2 in advanced cancer: Significant immunological modulation without toxicity (abstract). Proc Annu Meet Am Assoc Cancer Res 1991;32: A1463.
80 Eggermont AM, Goey SH, Slingerland R, Jansen RL, Oosterom R, Bolhuis RL, Stoter G: Clinical and immunological evaluation of intrapleural (ipl) interleukin-2 (IL-2) in malignant pleural mesothelioma: A phase I–II study (abstract). Proc Annu Meet Am Assoc Cancer Res 1991;32:A1228.
81 Israel L, Boaziz C, Moliard M, Morere JF, Breau JL: Phase II study of interleukin-2 in 18 patients with advanced gastrointestinal tract cancers (abstract). Proc Annu Meet Am Soc Clin Oncol 1991;10:A421.
82 Matijssen V, de Mulder PH, Schornagel JH, Verweij J, Van den Broek P, Galazka A, Roy S, Ruiter DJ: Clinical and immunopathological results of a phase II study of perilymphatically injected recombinant interleukin-2 in locally far advanced, nonpretreated head and neck squamous cell carcinoma. J Immunother 1991; 10:63.

83 Mertens WC, Bramwell VH, Lala PK: Continuous indomethacin and ranitidine with interleukin-2 in advanced renal carcinoma and melanoma (abstract). First Int Congr Biological Response Modifiers, Toronto, Feb 1991, A50.
84 Meyers JJ, Paradise C, Scudder SA, Goodman G, Konrad M: A phase I study including pharmacokinetics of polyethylene glycol conjugated interleukin-2. Pharmacol ther 1991;49:307.
85 Perez EA, Scudder SA, Meyers FA, Tanaka MS, Paradise C, Gandara DR: Weekly twenty-four hour continuous infusion interleukin-2 for malignant melanoma and renal cell carcinoma: A phase I study. J Immunother 1991;10:57.
86 Poo WJ, Fynan T, Davis C, Glynn S, Durivage H, Todd M: High-dose recombinant interleukin-2 alone in patients with metastatic renal cell carcinoma (abstract). Proc Annu Meet Am Soc Clin Oncol 1991;10:A557.
87 Velotti F, Stoppacciaro A, Ruco L, Tubaro A, Pettinato A, Morrone S, Napolitano T, Bossola PC, Franks CR, Palmer P: Local activation of immune response in bladder cancer patients treated with intraarterial infusion of recombinant interleukin-2. Cancer Res 1991;51:2456.
88 Clamon G, Ozer H, Herndon J, Perry M, Scalzo A, Green MR: Activity of interleukin-2 (IL-2) in patients (pts) with extensive small-cell lung cancer (abstract). Proc Annu Meet Am Soc Clin Oncol 1992;11A1057.
89 Escudier B, Rossi JF, Ravaud A, Douillard JY, Negrier S, Baume D, Dorval T, Chevreau C, Mignot L, Pein F: French experience of high-dose IL-2 on a two-days-a-week schedule in metastatic renal cell carcinoma: A multicentric study (abstract). Proc Annu Meet Am Soc Clin Oncol 1992;11:A651.
90 Gore ME, Riches P, MacLennan KA, O'Brien M, Moore J, Dadian G, Lorentzos A, Garth R, Moskovic E, Archer D: IA interleukin-2 (IL-2) in squamous cell carcinoma (SCC) of the head and neck (abstract). Proc Annu Meet Am Soc Clon Oncol 1992;22:A814.
91 Palmer PA, Philip T, Negrier S, Oskam R, Vinke J, Evers P, Becker L, Loriaux E, Franks CR, Kirchner: A comparison of 2 modes of administration of recombinant interleukin-2 (RIL-2, Proleukin) for patients with advanced renal cell cancer (RCC): Continuous iv infusion (CIV) vs. bolus sc administration (abstract). Proc Annu Meet Am Soc Clin Oncol 1992;11:A617.
92 Sleijfer DT, Janssen RAJ, Buter J, de Vries EG, Willemse PH, Mulder NH: Phase II study of subcutaneous interleukin-2 in unselected patients with renal cell cancer on an outpatient basis. J Clin Oncol 1992;10:1119.
93 Soiffer RJ, Murray C, Ritz J: Selective expansion and activation of NK cells and IL-2R positive T cells with combined low-dose continuous infusion and bolus IL-2 (abstract). Proc Annu Meet Am Assoc Cancer Res 1992;33:A1469.
94 Sorio R, Galligioni E, Sacco C, Morassut S, Freschi A, Quaia M, Spada A, Favaro D, Santarosa M, Boccalon M: Dose level and response in 30 patients (pts) with renal cell cancer (rcc) treated with recombinant interleukin-2 (RIL-2) (abstract). Proc Annu Meet Am Soc Clin Oncol 1992;11:A658.
95 Truitt RL, Piaskowski V, Kerchner P, McOlash L, Camitta BM, Casper JT: Immunological evaluation of pediatric cancer patients receiving recombinant interleukin-2 in a phase I trial. J Immunother 1992;11:274.
96 West WH, Tauer KW, Yannelli JR, Marshall GD, Orr DW, Thurman GB, Oldham RK: Constant-infusion recombinant interleukin-2 in adoptive immunotherapy of advanced cancer. N Engl J Med 1987;316:898–905.
97 Rosenberg SA, Packard BS, Aebersold PM, Solomon D, Topalian SL, Toy ST, Simon P, Lotze MT, Yang JC, Seipp CA: Use of tumor-infiltrating lymphocytes and interleukin-2 in the immunotherapy of patients with metastatic melanoma. N Engl J Med 1988;319: 1676–1680.
98 Dutcher JP, Creekmore S, Weiss GR, Margolin K, Markowitz AB, Roper M, Parkinson D, Ciobanu N, Fisher RI, Boldt DH: A phase II study of interleukin-2 and lymphokine-activated killer cells in patients with metastatic malignant melanoma. J Clin Oncol 1989;7: 477–485.
99 Hawkins MJ: PPO Updates iL-2/LAK. Principles Pract Oncol 1989;3:1–14.
100 Koretz MJ, Murray DR, Graham SD, Lawson DH, York RM, Sell KM: Randomized study of interleukin-2 (IL-2) alone versus IL-2 plus lymphokine activated killer cells for treatment of melanoma and renal cell cancer (abstract). 42nd Annu Cancer Symp Soc Surg Oncol, Orlando, Mar 1989, p 170.
101 Margolin KA, Rayner AA, Hawkins MJ, Atkins MB, Dutcher JP, Fisher RI, Weiss GR, Doroshow JH, Jaffe HS, Roper M: Interleukin-2 and lymphokine activated killer cell therapy of solid tumors: Analysis of toxicity and management guidelines. J Clin Oncol 1989;7:486–489.
102 Negrier S, Philip T, Stoter G, Fossa SD, Janssen S, Iacone A, Cleton FS, Eremin O, Israel L, Jasmin C: Interleukin-2 with or without LAK cells in metastatic renal cell carcinoma: A report of a European multicenter study. Eur J Cancer Clin Oncol 1989; 25(suppl 3):521–528.
103 Paciucci PA, Holland JF, Glidewell O, Odchimar R: Recombinant interleukin-2 continuous infusion and adoptive transfer of recombinant interleukin-2 activated cells in patients with advanced cancer. J Clin Oncol 1989;7:869–878.
104 Stahel RA, Sculie J, Jost LM, Delforge A, Bron D, Gmur J, Oelz O, Sauter C, Stryckmans P, Klastersky J: Tolerance and effectiveness of recombinant interleukin-2 [r-met Hu IL-2(ala 125)] and lymphokine-activated killer cells in patients with metastatic solid tumors. Eur J Cancer Clin Oncol 1989;25: 965–972.
105 Thompson JA, Lee DJ, Lindgren CG, Benz LA, Collins C, Shuman WP, Levitt D, Fefer A: Influence of schedule of interleukin-2 administration on therapy with interleukin-2 and lymphokine activated killer cells. Cancer Res 1989;49:235–240.
106 Dutcher JP, Gaynor ER, Boldt DH, Doroshow JH, Bar MH, Sznol M, Mier J, Sparano J, Fisher RI, Weiss G: A phase II study of high dose continuous infusion interleukin-2 with lymphokine-activated killer cells in patients with metastatic melanoma. J Clin Oncol 1991;9:641–648.
107 Hanson J, Petit R, Michalak M: Maximum tolerated dose (MTD) of IV continuous infusion )IVCI) interleukin-2 (IL-2) and lymphokine activated killer (LAK) cells (abstract). Proc Annu Meet Am Soc Clin Oncol 1990;9: A735.
108 Parkinson DR, Fisher RI, Rayner AA, Paietta E, Margolin KA, Weiss GR, Mier JW, Sznol M, Gaynor ER, Bar MH: Therapy of renal cell carcinoma with interleukin-2 and lymphokine-activated killer cells: Phase II experience with a hybrid bolus and continuous infusion interleukin-2 regimen. J Clin Oncol 1990;8: 1630–1636.
109 Steis RG, Urba WJ, VanderMolen LA, Bookman MA, Smith JW II, Clark JW, Miller RL, Crum ED, Beckner SK, McKnight JE: Intraperitoneal lymphokine-activated killer cell and interleukin-2 therapy for malignancies limited to the peritoneal cavity. J Clin Oncol 1990;8:1618–1629.
110 Usui A: Study on adoptive immunotherapy in patients with renal cell carcinoma. II. Plasmapheresis with adoptive immunotherapy using LAK cells and IL-2. Jpn J Urol 1990;81: 1058–1064.
111 Dillman RO, Oldham RK, Barth NM, Cohen RJ, Minor DR, Birch R, Yannelli JR, Maleckar JR, Sferruzza A, Arnold J: Continuous interleukin-2 and tumor-infiltrating lymphocytes as treatment of advanced melanoma. A National Biotherapy Study Group trial. Cancer 1991;68:1–8.
112 Han FG: Treatment of advanced liver cancer by autologous and/or homologous LAK cells combined with human natural IL-2. Chung Hua Chung Liu Tsa Chih 1991;13:145–148.
113 Hayes RL, Koslow M, Hiesiger EM, Hochster H, Hymes K, Moore E, Pierz DM, Wise A, Ransohoff J: Biologic response to intracavitary interleukin-2/lymphokine activated killer (LAK) cells in the treatment of primary malignant brain tumors. Dev Oncol 1991;66: 225–227.
114 Foon KA, Walther PJ, Bernstein ZP, Vaickus L, Rahman R, Watanabe H, Sweeney J, Park J, Vesper D, Russel D: Renal cell carcinoma treated with continuous-infusion interleukin-2 with ex vivo-activated killer cells. J Immunother 1992;11(3):184–190.
115 Weiss GR, Margolin KA, Aronson FR, Sznol M, Atkins MB, Dutcher JP, Gaynor ER, Boldt DH, Doroshow JH, Bar MH: A randomized phase II trial of continuous infusion interleukin-2 or bolus injection interleukin-2 plus lymphokine-activated killer cells for advanced renal cell carcinoma. J Clin Oncol 1992;10:275–281.
116 Stötter H, Lotze MT: Human lymphokine activated killer activity: Role of IL-2, IL-4, and IL-7. Arch Surg 1991;126:1525–1530.

117 Creekmore SP, Longo DL, Urba WJ: The development of regimens for combination immunotherapy; in Rees RC (ed): The Biology and Clinical Applications of IL-2. Oxford, Oxford University Press, 1990, p 98.

118 Albertini MR, Sosman JA, Hank JA, Moore KH, Borchert A, Schell K, Kohler PC, Bechhofer R, Storer B, Sondel PM: The influence of autologous lymphokine-activated killer cell infusions on the toxicity and antitumor effect of repetitive cycles of interleukin-2. Cancer 1990;66:2457.

119 Rosenberg SA, Lotze MT, Yang JC, Topalian SL, Chang AE, Schwartzentruber DJ, Aebersold P, Leitman S, Linehan WM, Seipp CA, White DE, Steinberg SM: Prospective randomized trial of high-dose interleukin-2 alone or in conjunction with lymphokine-activated killer cells for the treatment of patients with advanced cancer. J Natl Cancer Inst 1993;85:622–632.

120 Melder RJ, Whiteside TL, Vujanovic NL, Hiserodt JC, Herberman RB: A new approach to generating antitumor effectors for adoptive immunotherapy using human adherent lymphokine-activated killer cells. Cancer Res 1988;48:3461–3469.

121 Andeesen R, Scheibenbogen C, Brugger W, Krause S, Meerpohl HG, Leser HG, Engler H, Lohr GW: Adoptive transfer of tumor cytotoxic macrophages generated in vitro from circulating blood monocytes: A new approach to cancer immunotherapy. Cancer Res 1990; 50:7450.

122 Ting CC, Hargrove ME, Henrich P: Anti-CD3 antibody-induced activated killer cells. Subsets of killer cells that mediate fast or slow lytic reactions. Immunol Invest 1990;19:347.

123 Curti B, Ochoa JA, Urba W: Phase I study of patients treated with anti-CD3 stimulated cells (T-AK) and IL-2: Comparison of bolus and infusional IL-2 regimens. Proc Am Soc Clin Oncol 1992;11:A823.

124 Parmiani G: An explanation of the variable clinical response to interleukin-2 and LAK cells. Immunol Today 1990;11:113.

125 Crowley NJ, Darrow TL, Quinn-Allen MA, Seigler HF: MHC-restricted recognition of autologous melanoma by tumor-specific cytotoxic T cells. Evidence for restriction by a dominant HLA-A allele. J Immunol 1991; 146:1692.

126 Fisher B, Packard BS, Read EJ, Carrasquillo JA, Carter CS, Topalian SL, Yang JC, Yolles P, Larson SM, Rosenberg SA: Tumor localization of adoptively transferred Indium-111 labeled tumor infiltrating lymphocytes in patients with metastatic melanoma. J Clin Oncol 1989;7:250.

127 Reynolds CW, Denn AC III, Barlozzari T, Wiltrout RH, Reichardt DA, Herberman RB: Natural killer activity in the rat. IV. Distribution of large granular lymphocytes (LGL) following intravenous and intraperitoneal transfer. Cell Immunol 1984;86:371.

128 Yang SC, Owen-Schaub L, Mendiguren-Rodriquez A, Grimm EA, Hong WK, Roth JA: Combination immunotherapy for non-small cell lung cancer – results with interleukin-2 and TNF-α. J Thorac Cardiovasc Surg 1990; 79:8–13.

129 Whitehead RP, Friedman KD, Clark DA: A phase I trial of subcutaneous interleukin-2 and interleukin-4. Proc Annu Meet Am Assoc Cancer Res 1992;33:A1381.

130 Rosenberg SA, Lotze MT, Yang JC, Linehan WM, Seipp C, Calabro S, Karp SE; Sherry RM, Steinberg S, White DE: Combination therapy with interleukin-2 and alpha-interferon for the treatment of patients with advanced cancer. J Clin Oncol 1989;7:1863–1874.

131 Figlin RA, Belldegrun A, Moldawer N, Zeffren J, deKernion J: Concomitant administration of recombinant human interleukin-2 and recombinant interferon alpha-2a: An active outpatient regimen in metastatic renal cell carcinoma. J Clin Oncol 1992;10:414–421.

132 Krigel RL, Padavic-Shaller KA, Rudolph AR, Konrad M, Bradley EC, Comis RL: Renal cell carcinoma: Treatment with recombinant interleukin-2 plus beta-interferon. J Clin Oncol 1990;8:460–467.

133 Margolin KA, Doroshow JH, Akman SA, Leong LA, Morgan RJ, Raschko J, Somlo G, Mills B, Goldberg D, Sniecinski I: Phase I trial of interleukin-2 plus gamma interferon. J Immunother 1992;11:50–55.

134 Taylor CW, Chase EM, Whitehead RP, Rinehart JJ, Neidhart JA, Gonzalez R, Bunn PA, Hersh EM: A Southwest Oncology Group phase I study of the sequential combination of recombinant interferon-gamma and recombinant interleukin-2 in patients with cancer. J Immunother 1992;11:176–183.

135 Redman BG, Flaherty L, Chou TH, Al-Katib A, Kraut M, Martino S, Chen B, Kaplan J, Valdivieso M: A phase I trial of recombinant interleukin-2 with recombinant interferon-gamma in patients with cancer. J Clin Oncol 1990;8:1269–1276.

136 Viens P, Blaise D, Stoppa AM, Brandely M, Baume D, Olive D, Resbeut M, Delpero JR, Lopez M, Aubert C: Interleukin-2 in association with increasing doses of interferon-gamma in patients with advanced cancer. J Immunother 1992;11:218–224.

137 Smith KA: Interleukin-2: Inception, impact, and implications. Science 1988;240:1169.

138 Fidler IJ, Heicappell R, Saiki I, Grutter MG, Horisberger MA, Nuesch J: Direct antiproliferative effects of recombinant human interferon alpha. B/D hybrids on human tumor cell lines. Cancer Res 1987;97:2020.

139 Shiiba K, Suzuki R, Kawakami K, Ohuchi A, Kumagai K: Interleukin-2 activated killer cells: Generation in collaboration with interferon gamma and its suppression in cancer patients. Cancer Immunol Immunother 1986;21:119–128.

140 Atzpodien J, Korfer A, Palme PA, Franks CR, Poliwoda H, Kirchner H: Treatment of metastatic renal cell cancer patients with recombinant subcutaneous human interleukin-2 and interferon-alpha. Ann Oncol 1990;1: 377–378.

141 Bajorin DF, Chapman PB, Wong G, Coit DG, Kunicka J, Dimaggio J, Cordon-Cardo C, Urmacher C, Dantes L, Templeton MA: Phase I evaluation of a combination of monoclonal antibody R24 and interleukin 2 in patients with metastatic melanoma. Cancer Res 1990;50:7490–7495.

142 Atzpodien J, Kirchner H: The out-patient use of recombinant human interleukin-2 and interferon alfa-2B in advanced malignancies. Eur J Cancer 1991;27(suppl 4):S88–S91.

143 Fiorentino B, Amatetti C, DiStefano P, Giuliani C, Tinari N, Natoli C, Garufi C, Iacobelli S: Weekly sequential administration of interferon alpha-2B and interleukin-2 in patients with advanced malignancies. Proc Annu Meet Am Soc Clin Oncol 1992;11: A835.

144 Ziegler LD, Palazzolo P, Cunningham J, Janus M, Itoh K, Hayakawa K, Hellstrom I, Hellstrom KE, Nicaise C, Dennin R: Phase I trial of murine monoclonal antibody L6 in combination with subcutaneous interleukin-2 in patients with advanced carcinoma of the breast, colorectum, and lung. J Clin Oncol 1992;10:1470–1478.

145 Ettinghausen SE, Puri RK, Rosenberg SA: Increased vascular permeability in organs mediated by the systemic administration of LAK cells and recombinant interleukin-2 in mice. J Natl Cancer Inst 1988;80:177–188.

146 Lee RE, Lotze MT, Skibber JM, Tucker E, Bonow RO, Ognibene FP, Carrasquillo JA, Shelhamer JH, Parrillo JE, Rosenberg SA: Cardiorespiratory effects of immunotherapy with interleukin-2. J Clin Oncol 1989;7:7.

147 Mier JW, Vachino G, van der Meer JW, Numerof RP, Adams S, Cannon JG, Bernheim HA, Atkins MB, Parkinson DR, Dinarello CA: Induction of circulating tumor necrosis factor (TNF-alpha) as the mechanism for the febrile response to interleukin-2 (IL-2) in cancer patients. J Clin Immunol 1988;8: 426.

148 Fisher B, Keenan AM, Garra BS, Steinberg SM, White DE, DiBisceglie AM, Hoofnagle JH, Yolles P, Rosenberg SA, Lotze MT: Interleukin-2 induces profound reversible cholestasis: A detailed analysis in treated cancer patients. J Clin Oncol 1989;7:1852–1862.

149 Atkins MB, Mier JW, Parkinson DR, Gould JA, Berkman EM, Kaplan MM: Hypothyroidism after treatment with interleukin-2 and lymphokine activated killer cells. N Engl J Med 1988;318:1557–1563.

150 Gaspari AA, Lotze MT, Rosenberg SA, Stern JB, Katz SI: Dermatologic changes associated with interleukin-2 administration. JAMA 1987;258:1624.

151 Heslop HE, Gottlieb DJ, Bianchi AC, Meager A, Prentice HG, Mehta AB, Hoffbrand AV, Brenner MK: In vivo induction of gamma interferon and tumor necrosis factor by interleukin-2 infusion following intensive chemotherapy or autologous marrow transplantation. Blood 1989;74:1374.

152 Numerof RP, Aronson FR, Mier JW: Interleukin-2 stimulates the production of interleukin-1 alpha and interleukin-2 beta by human peripheral blood mononuclear cells. J Immunol 1988;141:4250.

153 Ochoa JB, Curt B, Peitzman AB, Simmons RL, Billiar TR, Hoffman R, Rault R, Longo DL, Urba WJ, Ochoa AC: Increased circulating nitrogen oxides after human tumor immunotherapy: Correlation with toxic hemodynamic changes. J Natl Cancer Inst 1992;84: 864.

154 Hibbs JB Jr, Westenfelder C, Traintor R, Vavrin Z, Kablitz C, Baranowski RL, Ward JH, Menlove RL, McMurry MP, Kushner JP: Evidence for cytokine inducible nitric oxide synthesis from *L*-arginine in patients receiving interleukin-2 therapy. J Clin Invest 1992; 89:867.

155 Fraker DL, Langstein HN, Norton JA: Passive immunization against tumor necrosis factor partially abrogates interleukin-2 toxicity. J Exp Med 1989;170:1015.

156 Oppenheim MH, Whiteside T, Bryant J, Lotze MT: Inhibition of tumor necrosis factor by pentoxifylline may partially reduce dose-limiting toxicities of interleukin-2 therapy; protocol in progress.

157 Borden EC, Schlom J: Williamsburg conference on biological and immunological treatments for cancer, 1992. J Natl Cancer Inst 1993;85:1288–1292.

158 Lotze MT, Oppenheim MH: Interleukin-2 and pentoxifyllin therapy of cancer patients. University of Pittsburgh, protocol in progress.

159 Interleukin-2 and *n*-monomethyl-*l*-arginine (NMMA) therapy in the treatment of advanced cancer. MD Anderson Cancer Hospital, protocol in progress.

160 Oppenheim MH, Leder G, Rosenstein M, Shah N, Hoffmann R, Simmons RL, Lotze MT: Aminoguanidine administration decreases serum nitric oxide levels in animals treated with interleukin-2 (IL-2); submitted.

161 Fearon ER, Pardoll DM, Itaya T, Golumbek P, Levitsky HI, Simons JW, Karasuyama H, Vogelstein B, Frost P: Interleukin-2 production by tumor cells bypasses T-helper function in the generation of an antitumor response. Cell 1990;60:397.

162 Golumbek PT, Lazenby AJ, Levitsky HL, Jaffee LM, Karasuyama H, Baker M, Pardoll DM: Treatment of established renal cancer by tumor cells engineered to secrete interleukin-4. Science 1991;254:713.

163 Tahara H, Mueller GM, Ricordi C, Robbins PD, Lotze MT: Islet cell transplantation facilitated by gene transfer. Transplant Proc 1992; 24:2975–2976.

164 Lotze MT: Work in progress on IL-12 transduced fibroblasts and tumor cells. University of Pittsburgh.

Oncology 1994;51:170–176

*Saburo Sone*
*Takeshi Ogura*

Third Department of Internal Medicine, The University of Tokushima School of Medicine, Tokushima, Japan

# Local Interleukin-2 Therapy for Cancer, and Its Effector Induction Mechanisms

**Key Words**
IL-2
Malignant pleuritis
Local immunotherapy
Killer induction

**Abstract**
This paper reviews the effectiveness of local interleukin-2 (IL-2) therapy and its effector induction mechanisms in vivo. Local therapy with IL-2 and/or lymphokine-activated killer (LAK) cells is associated with far fewer side effects than systemic treatment. Local infusions of IL-2 into malignant pleural effusions and the peritoneal cavity induce LAK cells and secondary production of other cytokines responsible for up- or down-regulation of LAK activity. An understanding of the regulatory mechanism of local LAK induction in vivo may provide the rationale for a more effective therapeutic modality for cancer in humans.

## Introduction

In vitro coculture of unprimed lymphocytes and interleukin-2 (IL-2) for 4–6 days results in the generation of nonspecific cytotoxic cells, named lymphokine-activated killer (LAK) cells, with a wide antitumor spectrum [1]. There is encouraging evidence that systemic administration of IL-2/LAK cells results in partial regression of terminal-stage cancer [2]. However, systemic intravenous (i.v.) administration of IL-2 in a dose effective for treatment of cancer patients causes severe side effects, such as vascular leak syndromes, extensive fluid retention, and life-threatening cardiopulmonary stress [3]. Several alternative approaches based on modifications of timing and route of administration have been attempted to improve response rates and decrease toxic effects by administering LAK cells and IL-2 directly into the tumor-growing site. Local IL-2 therapy is also advantageous when analyzing its immunopharmacological and therapeutic efficacy. Representative reports with local IL-2 and/or LAK cell therapy are summarized in table 1. In this review, we address the efficacy of local IL-2 and/or LAK cell therapy and their killer induction mechanisms in vivo.

## Efficacy of Local IL-2 Therapy for Malignancy

*Control of Malignant Effusions*
Local IL-2 instillation for malignant effusions associated with lung or ovarian cancer can be expected to have an antitumor effect because of a close interaction between tumor cells and IL-2-inducible killer cells, and the prolonged retention of IL-2 in the pleural or peritoneal cavity [4, 5]. In a preliminary study, LAK cells were found to be induced in the effusions of responders who exhibited the disappearance of pleural effusions and cancer cells from

Saburo Sone
3rd Department of Internal Medicine
The University of Tokushima School of Medicine
Kuramoto-cho 3
Tokushima 770 (Japan)


0030–2414/94/0512–0170
$5.00/0

the effusions [4]. Serial cytological examinations of pleural effusions following the start of local IL-2 instillation revealed the disappearance of malignant cells in 26 (74%) of 35 evaluable lung cancer patients [6]. Survival curves of the 54 patients with malignant pleural effusions who had been treated with local IL-2 instillation are shown in figure 1. Survival rates of responders and nonresponders at 1 year after the treatment were 40 and 21%, and median survival periods were 270 and 106 days, respectively.

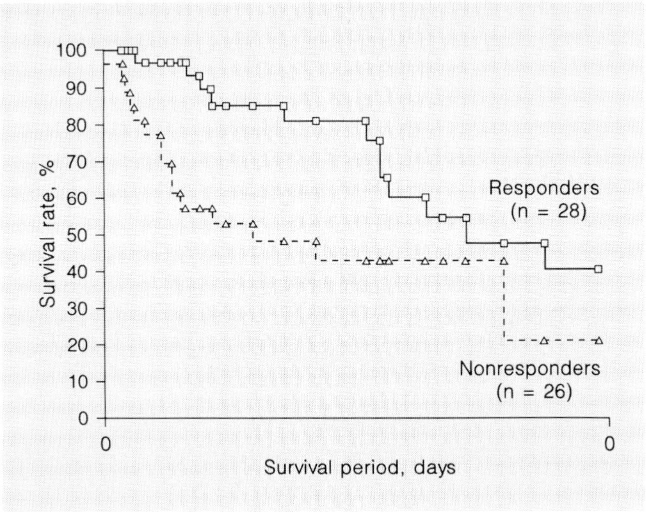


**Fig. 1.** Survival curves of evaluable patients with malignant pleural effusions. Recombinant IL-2 (250–1,000 U) was instilled into the pleural cavity for 5 to 33 days (mainly 14 days) through a double lumen trocar catheter.

**Table 1.** Efficacy of local therapy with IL-2 and/or LAK cells

| Cancer | IL-2/ LAK cells | Route of infusion | Antitumor effect | Reference |
|---|---|---|---|---|
| Recurrent glioblastoma | IL-2 LAK | intracavitary | PD: 8/13 cases 17 months after local therapy | Merchant et al. [12] |
| Malignant glioma | LAK-bispecific antibody | intracranial | no recurrence for 10–18 months in all 10 cases | Nitta et al. [16] |
| Malignant glioma | fresh lymphocytes | intracranial | R: 8/17 cases | Young et al. [11] |
| Meningeal gliomatosis and cancer | IL-2 LAK | intracisternal | R: 2/2 cases | Shimizu et al. [14] |
| Medulloblastoma in CSF | LAK | intrathecal | R: 3/6 cases | Okamoto et al. [15] |
| Malignant pleural effusion | IL-2 | intrapleural | R: 26/35 cases | Yasumoto and Ogura [6] |
| Pleural mesothelioma | IL-2 LAK | intrapleural | R: 2/2 cases | Yanagawa et al. [33] |
| Advanced malignancy | IL-2 | splenic artery | PR: 1/20 cases MR: 1/20 cases | Klasa et al. [24] |
| Liver metastases | IL-2 | splenic or hepatic | R: 2/28 cases | Mavligit et al. [21] |
| Malignant peritoneal effusion | IL-2 LAK | intraperitoneal | PR: 7/22 cases | Steis et al. [8] |
| Malignant peritoneal effusion | IL-2 | intraperitoneal | PR: 1/7 cases | Lotze et al. [3] |
| Malignant peritoneal effusion | IL-2 LAK | intraperitoneal | PR: 7/18 cases | Urba et al. [10] |
| Malignant peritoneal effusion | IL-2 LAK | intrapleural | R: 2/2 cases | Kamada et al. [7] |
| Ovarian cancer | IL-2 | intraperitoneal | PD: 4/7 cases NC: 3/7 cases | Chapman et al. [5] |
| Bladder cancer | IL-2 | intralesional | CR: 3/6 cases PR: 2/6 cases | Pizza et al. [18] |
| Bladder cancer | IL-2 | perfusion of bladder | CR: 1/5 cases | Huland and Huland [19] |
| Bladder cancer | IL-2 | intra-arterial | CR: 2/12 cases PR: 3/12 cases | Tubaro et al. [20] |

CSF = Cerebrospinal fluid; CR = complete response; MR = minor response; NC = no change; PD = progressive disease; PR = partial response; R = clinical response.

There are also successful clinical trials of local therapy with IL-2 plus LAK cells for malignancies limited to the peritoneal cavity [7–10]. For example, local instillation of IL-2 and LAK cells caused tumor regressions in 7 of 23 (30%) assessable patients [8]. Pharmacokinetic studies of intraperitoneal IL-2 administration revealed 10- to 100-fold higher concentrations of IL-2 in peritoneal fluid versus serum, and LAK activity was detectable in the peritoneal fluid until IL-2 administration was discontinued [10]. Nevertheless, no correlation was found between LAK cell lytic activity in peritoneal fluid and response to therapy [8].

*Local IL-2/LAK Cell Therapy for Brain Tumors*

There has been a clinical trial with recurrent glioma patients treated with autologous leukocyte infusions into the tumor bed or cystic cavity via an indwelling catheter [11]. The most significant result of this work was that about 8 of the 17 patients survived well beyond expectation. This finding was extended by several groups using local therapy with IL-2 and LAK cells [12–14]. For example, Merchant et al. [12] reported 9 patients with recurrent glioblastoma who received injections of autologous LAK cells and IL-2 into the brain tissue immediately surrounding the tumor cavity during craniotomy for subtotal tumor removal for 3 days after surgery, but the therapy was not effective in prolonging the survival of patients with a high postsurgical tumor burden.

Medulloblastomas are frequently seen in children and represent one-quarter of all pediatric brain tumors. They tend to disseminate along the cerebrospinal fluid (CSF) pathways. No therapeutic strategies are available to completely cure medulloblastoma with CSF dissemination. To overcome CSF dissemination of medulloblastoma, one-haplotype-identical LAK cells were transferred intrathecally in 6 patients who failed to respond to the initial treatment [15]. Three of them showed considerable responses to this local therapy, with improved neurological and cytological findings. One case was associated with hydrocephalus which might be due to a vascular leak syndrome or to the malabsorption of CSF by tumor dissemination and/or a high concentration of LAK cells.

To improve targeting of killer cells into tumor cells, Nitta et al. [16] constructed a bispecific antibody by chemically conjugating an anti-CD3 monoclonal antibody (MAb) to antiglioma MAb. Bispecific antibody induced more than 10- to 50-fold the original killer activity in LAK cells, and the antibody also conferred on the effector LAK cells high specificity for target cells like cytotoxic T lymphocytes (CTLs). With this specific targeting therapy, 4 out of 8 tumors regressed, and 4 remnant tumors were eradicated [16]. Remarkably, all patients are free from recurrence after 10–18 months of follow-up. Thus, local administration of LAK cells is likely to be more effective than systemic delivery, because it probably maximizes cell-to-cell contact between killer cells and glioma cells, and thus reduces the cell number required for tumor cell killing. Specific targeting therapy seems to be a promising approach to prevent the recurrence of postoperative glioma.

*Local IL-2 Treatment of Advanced Bladder Cancer*

Deep invasive bladder carcinoma seems also to be a good target for local IL-2 therapy, since the urinary bladder is one of the anatomic regions amenable to local and regional therapeutic control. Indeed, Bacillus Calmette-Guérin (BCG) perfusion of the bladder has been considered the most effective agent to reduce local recurrence rates after transurethral resection and induce regression of unresectable superficial neoplasms [17]. Encouraging preliminary results of locally administered IL-2 were reported in 1984 with perilesional injections of IL-2-rich supernatants in invasive bladder cancer [18]. Huland and Huland [19] demonstrated that local continuous perfusions of a high dose of IL-2 for 5 days induced local and systemic immunopotentiation. It should be noted that this local therapy was without any side effects.

An alternative approach consisting of continuous intra-arterial infusion of IL-2 has been attempted to treat low-stage transitional cell carcinoma of the bladder. When IL-2 was intra-arterially administered through the internal iliac artery in 12 patients with low-stage bladder cancer, complete and partial regression of the primary tumor was achieved in 5 of 12 patients, but no patient progressed [20]. A similar attempt was performed in patients with liver metastases by splenic or hepatic intra-arterial infusions of LAK or tumor-infiltrating lymphocytes, but clinical response was observed in only 2 of 28 patients [21]. Toxicities related to intra-arterial IL-2 infusion, comprising fever and hypotension, were observed in only 2 of 12 patients. A potential use of this regimen may be limited to patients at high risk for relapse and progression from superficial bladder cancer and/or patients with a partial response of minimal residual disease after systemic chemotherapy for locally advanced bladder cancer.

*Adverse Reactions Associated with Local IL-2 Therapy*

In general, acute systemic toxic effects such as hypotension, fever, chills, rash, nausea with vomiting, fluid retention and thrombocytopenia, seem to be less severe after local IL-2 therapy than during i.v. injection therapy of IL-2, and not dose-limiting. Nevertheless, local therapy with IL-2 and LAK cells is frequently associated with other side effects. For example, direct injection of LAK cells and IL-2 into the brain tissue seems to be safe, but symptoms of aseptic meningitis and increased intracranial pressure are displayed. Intraperitoneal therapy with IL-2 and LAK cells is associated with the undesirable side effect of abdominal pain secondary to ascites accumulation with significant weight loss, fever, nausea and vomiting, diarrhea and anemia [21]. On the other hand, intrapleural or intraperitoneal administration of IL-2 and/or LAK cells is frequently associated with development of local fibrosis, which limits the duration of effective therapy, particularly when repeated. Fibrosis results in an inability to drain effusions from the pleural or peritoneal cavity and to uniformly treat the entire surface of the cavity. Another problem is that the most common clotting abnormalities in cancer patients are elevated levels of fibrin/fibrinogen degradation products. Indeed fibrin is found in the fibrous stroma and surrounding tumor nodules and tumor cells, suggesting that fibrin deposition may protect tumor cells from destruction by cytotoxic cells through cell-to-cell contact. Recently, we observed a close correlation of the fibrinogen level in the plasma with its inhibitory effect on LAK-cell-mediated tumor cell killing in vitro, and that prevention of in vitro fibrin formation by an anticoagulant resulted in full expression of LAK-cell-mediated tumor cell killing [22]. These findings suggest that clinical treatment causing inhibition of fibrin formation in the pleural or peritoneal space might increase the cytotoxic effect of effector cells on cancer cells. These preliminary studies warrant the further exploration of modifications of this type of local therapy.

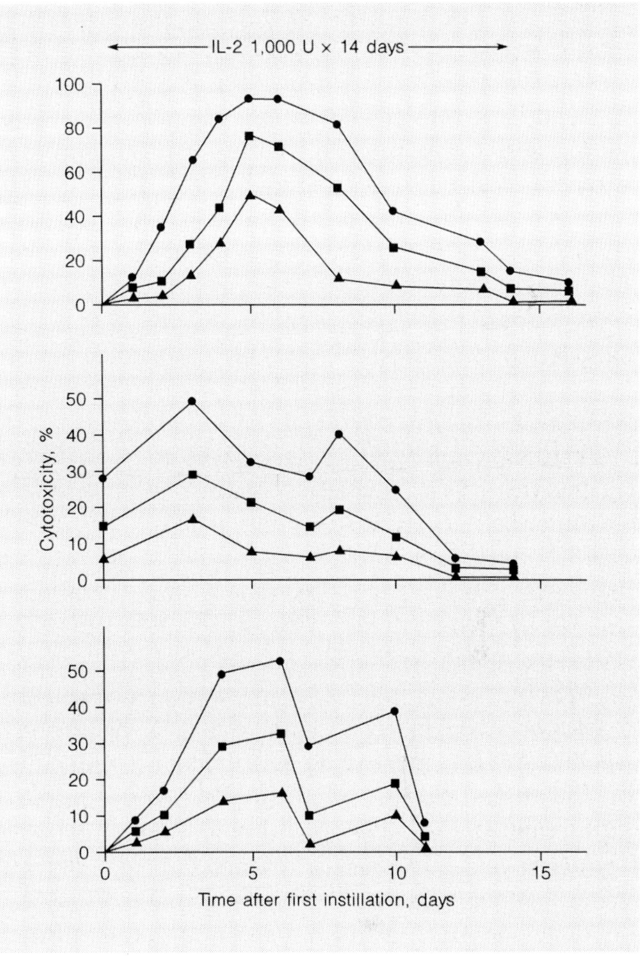


**Fig. 2.** In vivo induction of LAK cells in malignant pleural effusion by intrapleural daily injections of IL-2. Recombinant human IL-2 (1,000 U) was injected for 14 days, and LAK activity against Daudi cells was measured. Effector/target ratios: ● = 20; ■ = 10, and ▲ = 5.

## In vivo Induction of LAK Activity in Malignant Effusion

In an effort to stimulate in vivo LAK activity of patients with malignancy, recombinant IL-2 was administered by continuous 5-day splenic artery perfusion using the femoral approach. Splenic artery perfusion with IL-2 at relatively nontoxic doses resulted in significant in vivo generation of peripheral blood LAK cells, and it persisted at least 16 days after the cessation of treatment [23]. Such sustained LAK activity would not be expected with conventional high-dose i.v. IL-2 therapy. The kinetics of IL-2 decay may be altered in the spleen or a large pool of LAK and precursor cells may be generated which can then be released gradually into the peripheral blood.

It is also of much interest to examine whether the LAK activity of lymphocytes in malignant effusions can be induced by in vitro and in vivo IL-2 stimulation. Recently, daily intrapleural instillation of IL-2 was found to result in a disappearance of cancer cells with in vivo induction of tumor cytotoxic cells [4–6, 24]. In these studies, high LAK activity could be generated in cells of pleural effusions 3–5 days after the daily intrapleural instillations of IL-2. These findings strongly suggest that LAK precursors in malignant pleural effusions may be therapeutically useful, since cells harvested from malignant effusions can be allowed to grow in vitro in the presence of IL-2 in the hope of generating tumor-reactive populations of lymphocytes for adoptive immunotherapy. As shown in figure 2, kinetic study also showed that the LAK activi-

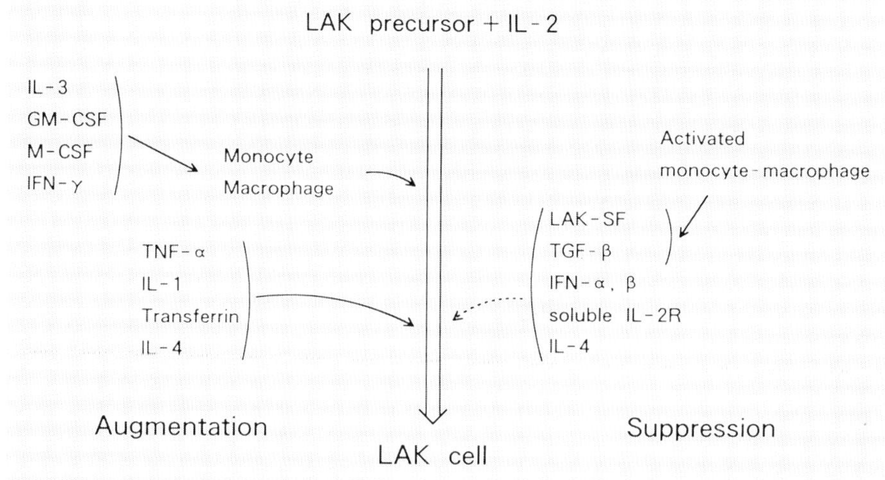


**Fig. 3.** Schema of regulatory mechanisms of LAK induction by IL-2. GM-CSF = Granulocyte-macrophage colony-stimulating factor; M-CSF = macrophage colony-stimulating factor; IFN = interferon; TNF = tumor necrosis factor; LAK-SF = LAK suppression factor; TGF = transforming growth factor.

ty in cells of malignant effusions was maximal 3–5 days after the local IL-2 therapy, but it decreased gradually, disappearing completely 15 days after the start of injections [24]. Disappearance of this LAK activity might be attributed to many cellular and humoral factors. One possibility is a rapid decay of the antitumor properties of the LAK cells. Indeed, when lymphocytes separated from pleural cells serially during local IL-2 therapy were restimulated for 4 days with optimal concentrations of IL-2 in vitro, the LAK activity gradually decreased after 7 days [24]. Another possibility is that it might be due to the disappearance of macrophages capable of up-regulating the LAK induction, because mature macrophages were susceptible to cytotoxicity by LAK cells [25]. We also found that macrophages isolated from malignant pleural effusions before IL-2 therapy augmented the IL-2-induced LAK activity of the autologous lymphocytes in effusions, like that of blood monocytes, but the up-regulatory properties of macrophages in the effusions decreased significantly after 10 days [24]. It is also possible that it might be due to a generation of inhibitory factors such as soluble IL-2 receptor (IL-2R) which was found to be released in large amounts from activated lymphoid cells. In fact, we also found that the level of soluble IL-2R increased during daily IL-2 injection into the pleural cavity [24]. There is accumulating evidence that LAK induction by IL-2 is up- or down-regulated by various humoral factors [26–30]. A schematic figure is given in figure 3. Thus, many factors may influence in vivo induction and maintenance of LAK activity.

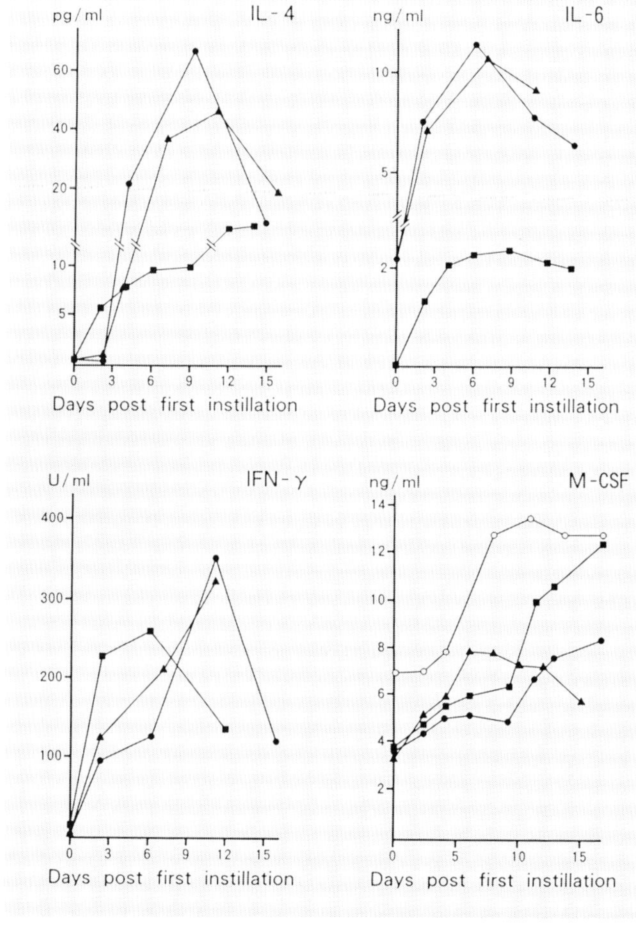


**Fig. 4.** Secondary production of cytokines in malignant pleural effusions of lung cancer patients by intrapleural daily injections of IL-2 (1,000 U) for 14 days.

## Secondary Induction of Cytokine Production after in vivo IL-2 Administration

IL-2 may induce peripheral blood mononuclear cells in vitro to produce secondarily a variety of cytokines such as tumor necrosis factor (TNF)-α, TNF-β, IL-1, IL-3, IL-5, granulocyte-macrophage colony-stimulating factor (GM-CSF) and interferon (IFN)-γ. It is important to examine whether in vivo instillations of IL-2 cause the secondary cytokine production. Indeed, i.v. infusions of recombinant human IL-2 were recently found to induce the production of IFN-γ, IL-5, IL-6, TNF-α, and CSFs in serum [31–34]. As shown in figure 4, intrapleural infusion of recombinant IL-2 into lung cancer patients with malignant pleural effusions caused an increase in the levels of IL-3, GM-CSF, macrophage colony-stimulating factor (M-CSF), IL-4, IFN-γ, IL-5, and IL-6 in pleural effusions, reaching maximal levels after 7–10 days. IL-4 down-regulates LAK induction, but augments LAK induction from human lymphocytes preactivated by IL-2 [26]. IFN-γ was also detected in the malignant ascitic fluid following intraperitoneal IL-2 infusion [10, 26]. In a parallel experiment, we also quantitated latent transforming growth factor (TGF)-β activity in cell-free effusion fluids before and during therapy with IL-2 alone or IL-2 and LAK cells, and found that latent TGF-.β activity increased during local IL-2 therapy [24]. In these studies, IFN-α, TNF-α and IL-1 were not detectable in the pleural effusions before and after local IL-2 therapy. This finding is in accordance with the previous observation showing no detectable production of TNF-α and IL-1β in the peritoneal fluid after local IL-2 injection [10]. The significance of the production of these secondary cytokines is not clear. Because in vitro studies previously showed that IL-4 and TGF-β down-regulated LAK induction [6, 35], the induction by IL-2 of secondary production of IL-4 and TGF-β may explain the mechanism of rapid decay of LAK activity. On the other hand, we have found that IL-3, GM-CSF, M-CSF and IL-5 seem responsible for the eosinophilia observed during the late course of IL-2 therapy [34]. Finally, understanding the regulatory mechanism of LAK induction may be important in providing a rationale for potentiation of IL-2-stimulated killer cells against cancer in humans. For this, further studies are required to elucidate the mechanisms of in vivo killer induction and its regulation through cytokine networks in humans.


## Acknowledgements

We are grateful to many colleagues for collaboration in the work mentioned in this review. This study was supported by a Cancer Research Grant from the Ministry of Health and Welfare of Japan.


## References


1 Grimm EA, Mazumder A, Zahng HZ, Rosenberg SA: Lymphokine-activated killer cell phenomenon. Lysis of natural killer-resistant solid tumor cells by interleukin 2-activated autologous human peripheral blood lymphocytes. J Exp Med 1982;155:1823–1841.
2 Rosenberg SA, Lotze MT, Muul LM, Chang AE, Avis FP, Leitman S, Linehan WM, Robertson CN, Lee RE, Rubin JT, Seipp CA, Simpson GC, White DE: A progress report on the treatment of 157 patients with advanced cancer using lymphokine activated killer cells and interleukin-2 or high dose interleukin-2 alone. N Engl J Med 1987;316:889–905.
3 Lotze MT, Chang AE, Seipp CA, Simpson C, Vetto JT, Rosenberg SA: High-dose recombinant interleukin-2 in the treatment of patients with disseminated cancer. Responses, treatment-related morbidity and histologic findings. JAMA 1986;256:3117–3124.
4 Yasumoto K, Miyazaki K, Nagashima A, Ishida T, Kuda T, Yano T, Sugimachi K, Nomoto K: Induction of lymphokine-activated killer cells by intrapleural instillations of recombinant interleukin-2 in patients with malignant pleurisy due to lung cancer. Cancer Res 1987; 47:2184–2187.
5 Chapman PB, Kolitz JE, Hakes T, et al: A phase I trial of intraperitoneal recombinant interleukin-2 in patients with ovarian cancer. Invest New Drugs 1988;6:179–188.
6 Yasumoto K, Ogura T: Intrapleural application of recombinant interleukin-2 in patients with malignant pleurisy due to lung cancer: A multi-institutional cooperative study. Biotherapy 1991;3:345–349.
7 Kamada M, Sakamoto Y, Furomoto H, Mori K, Daitoh T, Irahara M, Aono Y, Nii A, Yanagawa H, Sone S, Ogura T: Treatment of malignant ascites with allogeneic and autologous lymphokine-activated killer cells. Gynecol Oncol 1989;34:34–37.
8 Steis RG, Urba WJ, VanderMolen LA, Bookman MA, Smith JW II, Clark JW, Miller RL, Crum ED, Beckner SK, McKnight JE, Ozols RF, Stevenson HC, Young RC Longo DL: Intraperitoneal lymphokine-activated killer-cell and interleukin-2 therapy for malignancies limited to the peritoneal cavity. J Clin Oncol 1990;8:1618–1629.
9 Lotze MT, Custer MC, Rosenberg SA: Intraperitoneal administration of interleukin-2 in patients with cancer. Arch Surg 1986;121: 1373–1379.
10 Urba WJ, Clark JW, Steis RG, et al: Intraperitoneal lymphokine-activated killer cell/interleukin-2 therapy in patients with intra-abdominal cancer: Immunologic consideration. J Natl Cancer Inst 1989;81:602–611.
11 Young H, Kaplan A, Regelson W: Immunotherapy with autologous white cell infusions ('lymphocytes') in the treatment of recurrent glioblastoma multiforme: A preliminary report. Cancer 1977;40:1037–1044.
12 Merchant RE, Grant AJ, Merchant LH, Young HF: Adoptive immunotherapy for recurrent glioblastoma multiforme using lymphokine activated killer cells and recombinant interleukin-2. Cancer 1988;62:665–671.
13 Jacobs SK, Wilson DJ, Kornblith PL, Grimm EA: Interleukin-2 or autologous lymphokine-activated killer cell treatment of malignant glioma: Phase I trial. Cancer Res 1986;46: 2101–2104.
14 Shimizu K, Okamoto Y, Miyao Y, Yamada M, Ushio Y, Hayakawa T, Ikeda H, Mogami H: Adoptive immunotherapy of human meningeal gliomatosis and carcinomatosis with LAK cells and recombinant interleukin-2. J Neurosurg 1987;66:519–521.

15 Okamoto Y, Shimizu K, Tamura K, Miyao Y, Yamada M, Matsui Y, Tsuda N, Takimoto H, Hayakawa T: An adoptive immunotherapy of patients with medulloblastoma by lymphokine-activated killer cells (LAK). Acta Neurochir 1988;94:47–52.
16 Nitta T, Sato K, Yagita H, Okumura K, Ishii S: Preliminary trial of specific targeting therapy against malignant glioma. Lancet 1990;335: 368–371.
17 Lamm DL: Bacillus Calmette-Guerin immunotherapy for bladder cancer. J Urol 1985;134: 40–47.
18 Pizza GC, Severini G, Menniti D, et al: Tumor regression after intralesional injection of interleukin-2 (IL-2) in bladder cancer: Preliminary report. Int J Cancer 1984;34:359–367.
19 Huland E, Huland H: Local continuous high dose interleukin 2: A new therapeutic model for the treatment of advanced bladder cancer. Cancer Res 1989;49:5469–5474.
20 Tubaro A, Velotti F, Stoppacciaro A, Santoni A, Vicentini C, Bossola PC, Galassi P, Pettinato T, Morrone S, Napolitano T, Frati L, Ruco L, Franks CR, Palmer PA, Pourreau CN, Miano L: Continuous intra-arterial administration of recombinant interleukin-2 in low-stage bladder cancer. Cancer 1991;68:56–61.
21 Mavligit GM, Zukiwski AA, Gutterman JU, Salem P, Charnsangavej C, Wallace S: Splenic versus hepatic artery infusion of interleukin-2 in patients with liver metastases. J Clin Oncol 1990;8:319–324.
22 Atagi S, Sone S, Fukuta K, Ogura T: Inhibition by fibrin coagulation of lung cancer cell destruction by human interleukin-2-activated killer cells. Jpn J Cancer Res 1992;83:1088–1094.
23 Klasa RJ, Silver HKB, Kong S: In vivo induction of lymphokine-activated killer cells by interleukin-2 splenic artery perfusion in advanced malignancy. Cancer Res 1990;50: 4906–4910.
24 Yanagawa H, Sone S, Nii A, Fukuta K, Nakanishi M, Maeda K, Honda M, Ogura T: Lymphokine activated killer induction and its regulation by macrophages in malignant pleural effusions. Jpn J Cancer Res 1989;80:1220–1227.
25 Sone S, Inamura N, Singh SM, Okubo A, Yanagawa H, Nakanishi M, Ogura T: Killing of alveolar macrophages and of monocytes that have responded to granulocyte-macrophage colony-stimulating factor by human lymphokine-activated killer cells. Jpn J Cancer Res 1989;80:662–669.
26 Sone S, Yanagawa H, Nii A, Ogura T: Induction of interleukin 2-activated killer effector activity and its regulatory mechanism. Gann Monogr Cancer Res 1993;40:81–93.
27 Sone S, Munekata M, Nakamura A, Sugihara K, Nii A, Ogura T: Characterization and kinetics of a new monokine responsible for suppression of induction of lymphokine (IL-2)-activated killer activity. Cancer J 1991;4:89–96.
28 Sone S, Utsugi T, Nii A, Ogura T: Differential effects of recombinant interferons α, β, and γ on induction of human lymphokine (IL-2)-activated killer activity. J Natl Cancer Inst 1988; 80:425–431.
29 Sone S, Utsugi T, Nii A, Ogura T: Effects of human alveolar macrophages on the induction of lymphokine (IL-2)-activated killer cells. J Immunol 1987;139:29–34.
30 Nakamura A, Sone S, Nabioullin R, Sugihara K, Munekata M, Nii A, Ogura T: Augmentation by transferrin of IL-2-inducible killer activity and perforin production in DC8+ T cells. Clin Exp Immunol 1993;92:174–179.
31 Yanagawa S, Sone S, Munekata M, Ogura T: Identification of interleukin-6 in malignant pleural effusions and its augmentation by intrapleural instillation of interleukin-2. Clin Exp Immunol 1992;88:207–212.
32 Sone S, Nakanishi M, Ohmoto Y, Yanagawa H, Ogura T: Macrophage colony-stimulating factor activity in malignant pleural effusions: Its augmentation by intrapleural interleukin-2. Chest 1991;99:377–381.
33 Yanagawa H, Sone S, Fukuta K, Nishioka Y, Ogura T: Local adoptive immunotherapy using lymphokine-activated killer cells and interleukin-2 against malignant pleural mesothelioma: Report of two cases. Jpn J Clin Oncol 1991;21: 377–383.
34 Nakamura Y, Ozaki T, Yanagawa H, Yasuoka S, Ogura T: Eosinophil colony-stimulating factor induced by administration of interleukin-2 into the pleural cavity of patients with malignant pleurisy. Am J Respir Cell Mol Biol 1990; 3:291–300.
35 Grimm EA, Crump W III, Durett A, Hester JP, LagooDeenadalayan S, Owen-Schaub LB: Transforming growth factor beta (TGFβ) inhibits the in vitro induction of lymphokine-activated killing activity. Cancer Immunol Immunother 1988;27:53–58.

Oncology 1994;51:177–188

J.S. Cebon
G.J. Lieschke

Ludwig Institute for Cancer Research,
Melbourne Tumour Biology Branch,
Royal Melbourne & Austin Hospitals,
Melbourne, Vic., Australia

# Granulocyte-Macrophage Colony-Stimulating Factor for Cancer Treatment

**Key Words**
Granulocyte-macrophage colony-stimulating factor
High-dose chemotherapy
Bone marrow transplantation
Peripheral blood progenitor cells
Myeloid leukemia

**Abstract**
In the 5 years since granulocyte-macrophage colony-stimulating factor (GM-CSF) was first tested clinically, a number of different strategies for its use have been evaluated in patients with malignant disease. These include using GM-CSF to support standard and high-dose chemotherapy, to accelerate myeloid reconstitution following marrow transplantation, to mobilize peripheral blood progenitor cells into the circulation for harvesting and transplantation, and in combination with cycle-specific chemotherapy drugs to enhance their cytotoxicity to leukemic cells. Early results were encouraging and data from randomized studies are now being reported. These are enabling an assessment of the value of these strategies for GM-CSF use in the management of cancer.

## Introduction

The actions of granulocyte-macrophage colony-stimulating factor (GM-CSF) in early clinical studies have been reviewed recently [1–3]. Inevitably, comparisons arise between GM-CSF and granulocyte (G)-CSF. For many years these two molecules were not distinguished as separate components of the granulocyte-macrophage stimulating activity in unpurified tissue extracts and culture supernatants. It is now recognized that although they share many functions such as stimulating bone marrow colonies in vitro and activating mature granulocytes in a variety of functional assays, they are two distinct molecules encoded by different genes located on different chromosomes with no molecular homology, and each interacts with unique receptors [4]. Cells producing G-CSF and GM-CSF include monocytes, fibroblasts and endothelial cells. GM-CSF is also produced by activated T lymphocytes, cells not known to produce G-CSF [1, 4]. Each factor acts on immature myeloid progenitor cells and there is considerable overlap in the target cell populations. Nonetheless, GM-CSF acts on populations of more pluripotent cells giving rise to granulocyte macrophage colonies, and has some activity on progenitors capable of producing megakaryocytic and erythroid colonies [5]. In contrast, G-CSF acts primarily on a more lineage-restricted population of progenitor cells giving rise to granulocytes [6], although it can also synergize with growth factors acting on immature progenitor cells [7]. G-CSF is frequently detected in the serum of patients with fever and neutropenia [8], whereas GM-CSF is seldom detected in the circulation. It has been proposed that GM-CSF fulfills a role as a microenvironmental factor either at sites of inflammation or possibly also in the bone marrow stroma. G-CSF, being detected in the circulation, may well be a humoral 'neutropoietin' [8].

Dr. Jonathan S. Cebon, FRACP, PhD
Ludwig Institute Oncology Unit
Austin Hospital
Heidelberg, Vic. 3084 (Australia)


0030–2414/94/0512–0177
$5.00/0

Because of the similarities in action, both molecules have been evaluated for the same clinical applications. These include: (1) supporting standard-dose chemotherapy; (2) enabling dose-intensified chemotherapy to be administered; (3) accelerating hemopoietic recovery following bone marrow transplantation, and (4) enhancing the collection of peripheral blood progenitor cells (PBPC). Applications in the treatment of leukemia have also been tested including their use: (1) to accelerate myeloid recovery following cytotoxic therapy; (2) in combination therapy with cytotoxic drugs, and (3) as 'differentiation therapy'. From these studies there have been qualitative differences between these two molecules both in toxicity profiles, and for the cell populations stimulated by each [3]; however, direct comparative studies have not been performed.

The actions of GM-CSF which may distinguish it from G-CSF for anticancer therapy include: (1) stimulating macrophage-mediated antitumor activity by antibody-dependent cell cytotoxicity [9]; and (2) enhancing the immune response by increased class II antigen expression [10] or by eosinophil activation [11]. Despite these theoretical advantages in antitumor potential, there are little data from clinical trials demonstrating significant antitumor activity of GM-CSF [1]. Myeloid leukemic cells may differ in their response to these growth factors [12], and this may provide a rationale for either tailoring therapy or using combinations of CSFs in antileukemic treatment strategies.

## Phase I Studies

Phase I clinical studies for GM-CSF defined the maximum tolerated dose and evaluated the scheduling of GM-CSF administration either as a single agent or as an adjunct to chemotherapy. In summary, GM-CSF elevated neutrophil, eosinophil and monocyte counts [13–15], with variable effects on platelets and red cell counts. Occasional thrombocytopenia thought to be due to activation of the reticular endothelial system was observed [13]. Responding cell types increased in a dose-related manner [13, 16]. At dose levels >10 μg/kg eosinophilia contributed significantly to leukocytosis. GM-CSF enhanced the functional state of granulocytes and macrophages; for example, expression of adhesion molecules MO1 and Leu-M5 was increased [16–18] as was superoxide anion production by cells harvested from patients participating in GM-CSF studies [19, 20].

## GM-CSF following Standard-Dose Chemotherapy

GM-CSF was evaluated for patients receiving chemotherapy for sarcoma [21]. A first cycle containing GM-CSF had fewer days of neutropenia when compared to a non-GM-CSF-containing second cycle (3.5 compared to 7.4 days). The results of this study may have been influenced by cumulative effects of cytotoxic drug administration on the marrow. In another study in patients with a variety of tumors, GM-CSF-containing second cycles had less neutropenia, and this was associated with fewer days of fever and reduced antibiotic requirement [22]. In a small randomized study, three dose levels of GM-CSF were evaluated in patients with stage III or IV ovarian cancer, including comparisons with control patients receiving placebo. There was significantly reduced neutropenia in those patients receiving GM-CSF, particularly at the highest dose level (6 μg/kg/day). In addition, platelet counts were increased in GM-CSF-treated patients [23].

## GM-CSF for Chemotherapy Dose Intensification

It has been hoped that the hemopoietic growth factors would enable patients to benefit from the dose response relationship between chemotherapy delivered and chemosensitive tumors. Prior to formal phase II and III studies of truly dose-intense chemotherapy, some attempt has been made to redefine the toxicities of individual chemotherapeutic drugs and their combinations when supported with hemopoietic growth factors [24–26]. For some of these regimens the dose-limiting toxicities have continued to be hematological, whereas for others, nonhemopoietic toxicities have intervened. New maximum tolerated doses (MTDs) may need to be established for each dose-intense drug or combination supported with CSFs. Furthermore, cytokine combinations using synergizing CSFs and the use of marrow or PBPC are also being evaluated as methods of providing myeloid support. For each of these new supportive therapies, the toxicity profiles of intensified cytotoxic drug regimens will require reevaluation prior to phase II and III studies.

There are several approaches to dose intensification:

(1) To accelerate marrow recovery, GM-CSF can be administered after chemotherapy. Timing and dose appear to be important. From such studies [26–28], it appears that it is important to commence GM-CSF as soon as possible following chemotherapy, although cytotoxic drugs should probably be allowed to 'wash out' before stimulating myeloid proliferation.

(2) Certain schedules of GM-CSF given prior to chemotherapy may paradoxically increase myeloprotection and this may enable dose intensification. Mechanisms for this may include increasing the myeloid cell mass or inducing a quiescent state in the marrow by withdrawal of growth factor [27].

(3) Dose intensity may be increased by increasing the frequency of treatments with standard doses of cytotoxic agents. This has been evaluated for adriamycin with G-CSF [29], however when this was attempted for adriamycin and cyclophosphamide with GM-CSF support, cumulative myelotoxicity and prolonged thrombocytopenia occurred [30].

(4) GM-CSF may also be used as a component of therapy following the development of complications of neutropenia such as fever or infection. There are no published randomized studies evaluating this use of GM-CSF.

Table 1 shows a number of studies which have investigated dose-intense chemotherapy with GM-CSF support. Few of these studies have formally reestablished a MTD for single cytotoxic drugs or combinations, although the feasibility of delivering dose-intense schedules has been established and a number of these schedules are being advanced in further studies. Ongoing evaluation is required to determine the most appropriate way to deliver an increased intensity of chemotherapy. Whereas a single course of intensive chemotherapy (as is provided in marrow transplantation studies) may offer benefit in patients with chemosensitive malignancies, in other tumor types cyclical high-dose chemotherapy may be better. It therefore needs to be determined whether support with hemopoietic growth factors will enable both sustainable and cyclic high-dose chemotherapy to be delivered [43]. Although early randomized studies report reduced neutropenia and fever, it is more important to demonstrate clinical endpoints such as reduced infection rates and improved tumor response rates. This is less readily achieved. Longer-term evaluation is required to determine any improvements in disease-free or overall survival.

Formal dose intensification has been attempted in several of the studies shown in table 1 [24–26, 30, 42]. In most, however, intense regimens were chosen without a stepwise evaluation of the new MTD for these regimens. Many of the studies reported a reduction in neutropenia [24, 25, 27, 34–36, 38]. A significant reduction in the incidence of fever was reported in some studies [28, 36]. In contrast, the study of Hoekman et al. [30] found no decrease in the incidence of fever or infection in patients receiving GM-CSF. One randomized study has looked at the usefulness of GM-CSF as adjunctive therapy to high-dose chemotherapy. 182 patients treated for lymphoma with COP-BLAM chemotherapy were randomized to receive GM-CSF or placebo [40]. Those who received >70% of the planned GM-CSF had reduced incidence of infections. The early remission rate was higher in the subgroup of patients classified as 'high risk'. Most other reported studies performed comparisons with historical controls. Gurney et al. [34] performed a study with a crossover design enabling a comparison between patients receiving and not receiving GM-CSF, and in this small study no reduction in infections was observed. In some studies, infections were defined in terms of management practices rather than according to clinical or microbiological criteria, and this complicates the interpretation of the data.

Prolonged thrombocytopenia was noted in a number of studies [26, 30, 31, 33]. In some non-randomized comparisons, the opposite effect was noted, and GM-CSF appeared to support platelet counts [24, 28, 35]. Effects on platelet counts were variable and appeared to be dependent upon the chemotherapy regimen. Prolonged thrombocytopenia was reported as a reason for not being able to establish a new MTD for thio-TEPA [33]. Increasing the frequency of GM-CSF injections may improve its efficacy. When increased doses of carboplatin were administered together with cyclophosphamide (1 g/m$^2$), the dose could not be escalated beyond 300 mg/m$^2$ using a daily GM-CSF schedule (dose 20 µg/day). Further escalation to 700 mg/m$^2$ was possible when the GM-CSF dosage was changed to 10 µg/kg administered every 12 h [44].

It may be important to sustain dose intensity over a number of treatment cycles. Several studies report that GM-CSF does not abrogate cumulative myelotoxicity following multiple cycles of chemotherapy. Bishop et al. [26] showed the importance of the schedule of GM-CSF administration relative to chemotherapy administration. However, despite identifying an optimal schedule and increasing the frequency of the GM-CSF injections, dose-intense chemotherapy could not be supported beyond 3 cycles for patients with small cell lung cancer receiving double dose carboplatin and VP-16 supported with subcutaneous (s.c.) GM-CSF twice daily. In another study, adriamycin (90 mg/m$^2$) in combination with cyclophosphamide (1 g/m$^2$) could not be supported by GM-CSF because of cumulative myelotoxicity [30]. As a result, the cytotoxic drugs required dose reduction to 75 mg/m$^2$ and 750 mg/m$^2$, respectively, and despite this platelet and red blood cell transfusion support was necessary for some patients in later cycles. Similarly, carboplatin dose intensity [42] could not be sustained beyond 600 mg/m$^2$, and

**Table 1.** High-dose chemotherapy supported with GM-CSF

| Chemotherapy | | n | GM-CSF, μg/day | Observations | Reference |
|---|---|---|---|---|---|
| *Fixed high-dose chemotherapy, varied GM-CSF dose* | | | | | |
| Carboplatin | 1,200 mg/m² | 12 | 5–10/kg | prolonged TP and NP | 31 |
| Melphalan | 100 mg/m² | 23 | 250–750/kg | ↓NP | 32 |
| CYADIC | 5 days<br>3 days | 7<br>17 | 120–750/m² | high-dose chemotherapy supported | 27 |
| Thio-TEPA | 75 mg/m² | 13 | 5–10/kg | ANC supported; prolonged TP prevented; ↑ DI | 33 |
| Ifosfamide<br>Doxorubicin<br>Etoposide | 5 g/m²<br>50 mg/m²<br>120 mg/m² | 13 | 50–500/m² | ↓ NP; crossover design | 34 |
| Melphalan | 120 g/m² | 9 | 3–10/kg | ↓ NP; ↓ TP | 35 |
| Cyclophosphamide<br>VP-16<br>Cisplatinum | 2.5 g/m² × 2 days<br>500 mg/m² × 3 days<br>50 mg/m² × 3 days | 23 | 250–1,000/m² | ↓ 'cytopenias'; ↓ hospitalization | 36 |
| Escalated MVAC | | 32 | 120–250/m² | high-dose chemotherapy supported | 37 |
| Carboplatin<br>VP-16 | 100–200 mg/m² × 3 days<br>120–240 mg/m² × 3 days | 44 | 5–15/kg | cumulative myelotoxicity, especially TP | 26 |
| *Fixed high-dose chemotherapy, fixed GM-CSF dose* | | | | | |
| Cyclophosphamide | 7 g/m² | 15 | 5.5/kg | ANC supported; ↓ TP; ↓ infections | 28 |
| Mitoxantrone<br>Ara C | 10 mg/m² × 2 days<br>6 g/m² × 2 days | 23 | 250/m² | ↓ NP; ↓ stomatitis | 38 |
| Mitoxantrone<br>Ara C | 5 mg/m² × 5 days<br>6 g/m² × 3 days | 34 | 125/m² | ↓ NP; no effect on platelets or infections | 39 |
| COP-BLAM | | 182 | 400 | ↓ infections and hospitalization[1];<br>↑ tumor response (high-risk patients) | 40 |
| Adriamycin<br>Ifosfamide | 75 g/m²<br>5 g/m² | 47 | 250/m² | DI and dose interval maintained in some patients | 41 |
| *Chemotherapy dose escalation* | | | | | |
| Carboplatin<br>Cyclophosphamide | 225–700 mg/m²<br>1 g | 36 | 10/kg<br>every 2 h | ANC and platelets supported | 24 |
| Cyclophosphamide | 1.5–4.5 g/m² | 17 | 10/kg | ANC supported | 25 |
| Adriamycin<br>Cyclophosphamide<br>up to 7 cycles | 75–90 g/m²<br>750–1,000 g/m² | 18 | 250/m² | modest ↑ DI not sustainable because of cumulative myelotoxicity | 30 |
| A Carboplatin<br>Cyclophosphamide<br>B Carboplatin | 400–600<br>1,000<br>600 | 15<br><br>7 | 250/m² | ↑ DI of Carboplatin prevented by TP | 42 |
| Carboplatin<br>VP-16 | 100–200 mg/m² × 3 days<br>120–240 mg/m² × 3 days | 44 | 5–15/kg | cumulative myelotoxicity, especially TP | 26 |

CYADIC = Cyclophosphamide 750 mg/m², adriamycin 75 mg/m², dacarbazine 1,000 mg/m²; MVAC = methotrexate 30 mg/m², vinblastine 4 mg/m², doxorubicin 60 mg/m², cisplatin 100 mg/m²; COP-BLAM = cyclophosphamide + vincristine + prednisone + bleomycin + doxorubicin + procarbarzine; TP = thrombocytopenia as measured by various parameters chosen by individual investigators; NP = neutropenia; ANC = absolute neutrophil count; DI = dose intensification.

[1] For patients who received >70% of study medication.

**Table 2.** Hematologic and clinical effects of GM-CSF after myeloablative therapy

| Type of cancer | Number of patients, treatment/control | Study phase | Treatment regimen | GM-CSF dose µg/day | Hematologic effects[1], treatment/control | Clinical effects | |
|---|---|---|---|---|---|---|---|
| | | | | | | days of fever | days in hospital |
| *Myeloablative therapy followed by autologous marrow transplantation* | | | | | | | |
| Breast and melanoma [45] | 19/24 | I-II | HDCT | 2–30/kg | 16/19 | – | – |
| ALL, NHL [46] | 14/86 | I-II | TBI + HDCT | 15–240/m² | 14/25 | 8/12 | 29/41 |
| ALL [47] | 25/27 | I-II | TBI + HDCT | 16–256/m² | | – | – |
| HD [48] | 12/19 | I-II | HDCT | 100–400/m² | 18/25 | – | – |
| ALL, NHL, HD [49] | 65/63 | III | HDCT + TBI | 250/m² | 19/26*** | 8/8 | 27/33** |
| HD, NHL [50] | 36/33 | III | HDCT ± TBI<br>BM or PBPC or both | 10/kg | 12/16* | not stated | 27/27 |
| HD [51] | 12/12 | III | HDCT ± TNI | 10/kg | 16/27* | not stated | 32/40.5** |
| HD or NHL [52] | 29/29 | III | HDCT | 250/m² | 14/20*** | 8/6 | 24/25 |
| NHL [53] | 44/47 | III | HDCT | 250/m² | 14/21*** | not stated | 23/28* |
| ALL, NHL [54] | 79 | III | TBI + HDCT | 250/m² | 15/25*** | reduced bacterial infections | – |
| *Myeloablative therapy by allogeneic marrow transplantation* | | | | | | | |
| ALL, AML, CML, HD, NHL, other [55] | 45/93 | I-II | HCDT ± TBI | 30–500/m² | | | |
| | | | MTX | | 20/24** | 4/9** | 24/31* |
| | | | no MTX | | 14/19** | 9/8 | 33/36 |
| AML, ALL, CML, NHL [56] | 29/28 | III | HDCT ± TBI<br>T cell depleted | 5.5/kg | 15.8/19.9[2,*] | 11/13[2] | 42/43[2] |
| AML, ALL, CML, other [57] | 20/20 | III | HDCT ± TBI | 5.5/kg | 13/16 | increase | not stated |

For GM-CSF vs. placebo: * $p < 0.05$, ** $p < 0.01$, *** $p < 0.001$. NHL = Non-Hodgkin's lymphoma; HD = Hodgkin's disease; ALL = acute lymphoblastic leukemia; GC = germ cell tumor; AML = acute myeloid leukemia; CML = chronic myeloid leukemia; TBI = total body irradiation; TNI = total nodal irradiation; MTX = methotrexate; HDCT = high-dose chemotherapy; BM = bone marrow; PBPC = peripheral blood proliferative cells.

1 Days to ANC (or neutrophil count) $>0.5 \times 10^9$/l. Values are medians unless otherwise indicated.

2 Means.

after 2 or 3 cycles at this dose, delays or dose reductions were required because of prolonged cytopenias.

In summary, currently available reports have shown that GM-CSF probably confers a modest advantage to enable delivery of intensified chemotherapy. However, there is little evidence that any beneficial effects on neutrophils or platelet counts, which occur in early cycles of therapy, can be sustained. Some studies report modest benefit in terms of infection rates. Although an improved tumor response rate in high-risk patients with lymphoma has been reported, this observation requires confirmation, and it is too early to say whether or not support of standard or high-dose chemotherapy with GM-CSF results in any beneficial tumor-related outcome.

## Bone Marrow Transplantation

CSFs have been used to accelerate myeloid reconstitution following myeloablation for patients receiving autologous marrow, peripheral blood progenitor cells (PBPCs) or allogeneic bone marrow (table 2). In addition, CSFs have been used in patients with poor engraftment or graft failure. Accelerated myeloid reconstitution can reduce morbidity due to infection, thrombocytopenic bleeding, and by reducing mucositis. It is unlikely that CSFs will prevent the toxicities of conditioning regimens which involve nonhemopoietic organs such as veno-occlusive disease of the liver, or pneumonitis. In allogeneic marrow transplantation there has been a concern that GM-CSF may influence immune reconstitution since it has inherent immunomodulatory effects such as stimulating macrophage activation and antigen presentation [10]. Nonetheless, the theoretical effects on graft-versus-host disease (GVHD) may be balanced by the benefit resulting from reduced infection rates.

In early transplant studies, the dose of GM-CSF was investigated (table 2). The dose range chosen for later studies has been around 250 μg/m²/day or 5–10 μg/kg/day, a dose similar to that preferred for other indications. Intravenous (i.v.) administration has generally been chosen as the preferred route, either by short (2 h) or continuous infusion. Following marrow transplantation, the adverse effects of GM-CSF are more difficult to recognize because of the toxicities associated with the conditioning therapy, however, in some randomized studies [49, 50], no toxicity attributable to GM-CSF was seen in the setting of autologous transplantation. In allogeneic bone marrow transplantation, GM-CSF was reported to cause an increase in fevers resulting in increased use of empiric antibiotics [55].

A reduction in neutropenia was reported in several phase I and II studies [45, 46, 48]. Although reduced neutropenia did not achieve statistical significance in some of these studies, this may reflect study designs which investigated a range of GM-CSF doses. In reported randomized studies, a significant decrease in neutropenia has been consistently reported [49–51, 53]. Reductions in median time to an absolute neutrophil count (ANC) of 500/μl were from 26 to 19 days in patients with lymphoid malignancies [49], from 27 to 16 days in patients with relapsed Hodgkin's disease [51], from 16 to 12 days in patients with lymphoma receiving either marrow or PBPC [50], from 21 to 14 days, and 20 to 14 days and 28 to 15 days in patients receiving autologous marrow transplantation for non-Hodgkin's lymphoma [51, 52] or acute lymphoblastic leukemia [54]. Reduced neutropenia resulted in fewer days in hospital for patients receiving GM-CSF in 3/5 of these randomized studies. The median reduction was 6 [49], 5 [53] and 8.5 [51] days. Reduced neutropenia conferred benefit in infection rates in three studies [49, 50, 54], but this was not observed in the other studies. In the study of Nemunaitis et al. [49], there was a significant reduction of documented infections in the first 28 days (17 vs. 30%, $p = 0.01$). Similarly, days of i.v. antibiotics were reduced from 27 in control patients to 24 in patients receiving GM-CSF ($p = 0.009$). The median duration of febrile episodes was identical in each group and there was no difference in the number of infectious deaths. A reduction in infection rates was also reported in patients who were treated on a mixture of protocols, some of which included marrow purging or infusion of PBPC [50]. It is less certain that this reduction was due to GM-CSF, since the patient groups in this study were not well matched for purging (which delayed engraftment) or PBPC infusions (which reduced time to engraftment). The duration of severe neutropenia (ANC $<0.1 \times 10^9$/l) [52] was not reported in all studies, and only appeared to be reduced by 0 [52] to 1 [49] day. This modest reduction in the period at which there is greatest risk of bacterial infections may explain why there was no consistent reduction in documented infection rates in these studies. Effects on platelet and red blood cell transfusion requirements were less consistent, with only one study documenting a reduced requirement for platelet transfusions [51].

The toxicities attributable to GM-CSF following marrow transplantation have generally been mild. Capillary leak syndrome [52, 53] has been a problem in a minority of patients. Fever has been observed in some patients receiving GM-CSF following myeloablative therapy but prior to becoming frankly neutropenic [52]. GM-CSF did not appear to adversely affect disease-free survival in the patients who participated in these studies. Although the impact on infectious outcomes has been modest, days of hospitalization were reduced in the majority of these studies [49, 51, 53]. This provided substantial cost benefit for patients who received GM-CSF [51].

In allogeneic bone marrow transplantation, patients receiving GM-CSF had reduced neutropenia, days of fever and days of hospitalization [55]. In this nonrandomized dose escalation study, benefit was only seen in patients who were not receiving methotrexate as anti-GVDH prophylaxis. There did not appear to be an increased incidence of GVHD. A randomized study performed in 57 patients who received T-cell-depleted marrow demonstrated accelerated recovery to neutrophils $>0.5 \times 10^9$/l (mean: 4 days). This was not associated with a reduced number of infections or febrile episodes although there were fewer lethal infections in the GM-CSF-treated group (1/29 vs. 4/28) [56]. In another smaller randomized study [57], a 3-day difference in the rate of recovery of the neutrophil count did not translate into clinical benefit in terms of fever and infection. Indeed, fever caused by the study drug appeared to result in greater use of empiric antibiotics. In this study (which included patients with a prior diagnosis of myeloid leukemia) it was noteworthy that there was no effect on the leukemic relapse rate in the GM-CSF-treated group.

## Peripheral Blood Progenitor Cells

During the recovery phase which follows myelotoxic chemotherapy, myeloid progenitor cells are detected in increased numbers in the circulation [58]. This phenomenon also occurs following administration of GM-CSF whether or not it follows chemotherapy [59, 60], and with G-CSF [61]. Progenitor cell numbers in the circulation can increase by 10- to 100-fold. Using the granulocyte-macrophage colony-forming (CFU-GM) cell as an index of progenitor cell and repopulating cell dose, it has been proposed that to achieve adequate reconstitution, a dose of $30 \times 10^4$ CFU-GM cells/kg needs to be infused [62]. These cell quantities are obtainable from the peripheral blood using GM-CSF alone [59, 60]. This has resulted in the development of strategies which harvest peripheral PBPC for transplantation.

Advantages of this approach include: (1) obviation of the need for marrow harvest; (2) a potentially tumor-free source of progenitor cells when bone marrow is involved; (3) progenitor cell collection from patients with marrow damage precluding marrow harvest, such as that caused by radiotherapy. Further advantages have been demonstrated in clinical studies using these cells including (1) acceleration of multilineage myeloid reconstitution (i.e., consistent acceleration of platelet recovery and reduced red blood cell transfusion requirements in addition to leukocyte recovery, and (2) reduction in nonhematologic morbidity such as mucositis. Consequently, general supportive-care requirements and days in hospital can be reduced.

Approaches evaluated include either mobilizing PBPC using cytotoxic drugs followed by GM-CSF [63, 64], or mobilizing PBPC using GM-CSF alone [65, 66]. Using combinations of CSFs to mobilize PBPC may also improve progenitor yields [67]. Harvested PBPC can be used to augment marrow infusion [63, 68] or can be infused alone without bone marrow [64–66]. Similar strategies have been successfully adopted for G-CSF [69].

The clinical application of GM-CSF to mobilize progenitor cells was first reported in seven patients with non-Hodgkin's lymphoma [63]. These patients were treated with autologous bone marrow transplantation supplemented with PBPC which had been mobilized by high-dose cyclophosphamide followed by GM-CSF. The addition of GM-CSF to high-dose chemotherapy resulted in a 7-fold increase in the yield of progenitor cells obtained by cytopheresis [70]. The myeloid recovery in these patients was compared with that in a group of control patients who received PBPC mobilized with chemotherapy alone. The addition of PBPC to autologous marrow transplantation resulted in the rapid appearance of neutrophils (mean: 9.1 ± 0.9 days to reach an ANC of 500/µl). Platelet recovery (10.7 ± 2.6 days to 50,000/µl) was substantially faster than that which followed bone marrow transplantation alone. This may be because the PBPC infusions contained larger numbers of committed progenitor cells which were capable of generating mature cells in less time. Mucositis was also reduced and this may reflect accelerated neutrophil recovery [71].

Other studies have demonstrated that GM-CSF-mobilized PBPC can significantly reduce the times of myeloid reconstitution and hospizalization [64, 68]. In a group of 16 patients, compared with 29 historical controls, infusion of PBPC alone was compared with an identically treated group of patients who received a marrow transplant. The patients receiving PBPC had a significantly reduced time to neutrophil and platelet recovery, and reduced numbers of febrile days, platelet transfusions, hospital days and red blood cell transfusion requirements. A small subset of patients had poor engraftment and required prolonged support. These required the use of reserve marrow because of slow platelet engraftment, and in retrospect could be identified as those who appeared to have poor myeloid reserves [64].

To test whether or not mobilized progenitor cells could be used in patients who were unsuitable for bone marrow harvest because of prior marrow damage caused by radiotherapy and chemotherapy, twelve patients with Hodgkin's disease were transplanted with progenitor cells mobilized by either chemotherapy or GM-CSF [65]. Although patient numbers were small, the time to reconstitution of the neutrophil count and platelet counts were comparable whether progenitors were mobilized by chemotherapy or GM-CSF. The time range to ANC >500/µl was 9–26 days, and 4–43 days, respectively. The time range to platelets >20,000/µl was 17-'not reached' and 22–55 days for chemotherapy or GM-CSF-mobilized PBPCs, respectively. The reported follow-up was for 187+ and 257+ days. This study established that PBPCs alone could be used to attain engraftment even if extensive prior marrow damage had occurred, and that multilineage engraftment took place. Similar findings were reported in a group of heavily pretreated patients who received GM-CSF to mobilize progenitors [66]. An 8.5-fold increase in marrow-colony-forming units resulted, and sustained engraftment was obtained in 5 of 6 patients with a median of 28.5 days to ANC 500/µl and 39 days to platelets >20,000/µl.

The integrity of the progenitor cell pool appears to be important. Even though the progenitor cells from patients with damaged marrows can be used to sustain engraftment in these patients, times to reconstitution of counts were longer and yields were lower [65, 66]. Smaller numbers of CD34+ progenitor cells are mobilized in this group [67]. Not only does prior myelotoxic therapy appear to effect the yield of PBPC, so does extensive tumor infiltration. In one instance, extensive replacement of marrow with myeloma resulted in no GM-CSF-induced progenitor mobilization [66].

New approaches are being developed to optimize the yield of PBPC and thereby minimize the number of procedures which need to be performed. These include combining cytokines and cytotoxic drugs, and using combinations of cytokines such as GM-CSF and interleukin-3 (IL-3) or adding other early-acting growth factors. In vitro expansion of progenitor cells is also being investigated. Combining cytokines with chemotherapy appears to result in greater yields of assayable progenitors such as CFU-GM and multi-lineage progenitors (CFU-GEMM) [67]. The median yield of progenitors was increased by adding GM-CSF to VIP chemotherapy (VP-16, ifosfamide, cisplatinum) and increased further when IL-3 was added. The problem remains that CFU-GM and CFU-GEMM assays do not identify cells which are responsible for long-term myeloid reconstitution, and the numbers of these cells do not necessarily correlate well with each other or with CD34+ cell numbers [67]. The only real assay for repopulating cells at present is transplantation itself, and without cell-marking studies it is still unclear whether or not the long-term hemopoiesis comes from transplanted cells or from residual stem cells which may have survived conditioning therapy. Nonetheless, long-term hemopoiesis occurs following PBPC alone, with reported follow-ups ranging from 12 to 23 months [64, 65]. It seems likely that long-term marrow repopulating cells are included among those which are mobilized by GM-CSF.

In summary, GM-CSF administered either alone or following chemotherapy can mobilize sufficient progenitor cells to achieve sustained engraftment. Multilineage engraftment occurs earlier in patients receiving these cells than in those receiving marrow, and this is presumably because multilineage progenitor cells are mobilized even though in other regards GM-CSF is a lineage-restricted growth factor. The consequence of accelerated myeloid reconstitution is reduced toxicity and morbidity.

Are these approaches applicable for allogeneic bone marrow transplantation? To date, mobilization of progenitors for this purpose has not been reported. Several issues need to be resolved for this application to be considered. Firstly, there is the concern that infusion of lymphocytes in the mononuclear cell fraction may increase the risk of GVHD. Secondly, the ability of PBPC to sustain long-term engraftment in a foreign-marrow environment remains untested. Finally, GM-CSF has a spectrum of adverse effects which may occur in allogeneic donors. G-CSF, which has a more limited profile of adverse effects may be preferable for use in normal donors.

### GM-CSF for the Treatment of Leukemia

CSFs can be used in the treatment of leukemia either to accelerate myeloid recovery following chemotherapy, to induce differentiation of leukemic blast cells, or to enhance the toxicity of cell-cycle-specific drugs such as cytosine arabinoside. These approaches remain experimental and are not recommended for routine clinical use because the safety and value of administering CSFs to patients with myeloid malignancies has not been determined.

To evaluate the safety and efficacy of GM-CSF following induction therapy for acute myeloid leukemia, GM-CSF was administered to patients with a poor prognosis (>65 years of age or with relapsed disease). Thirty-two patients were administered a dose of 250 μg/m$^2$ i.v., following a biopsy which established bone marrow aplasia and contained fewer than 5% blasts [72]. GM-CSF resulted in a reduction in the time to neutrophil recovery (median 6 or 9 days depending on which chemotherapy regimen was used) when recovery was compared with a historical series of patients.

Accelerated myeloid recovery was associated with fewer early deaths and an improved complete response rate (50 vs. 32%). GM-CSF did not affect the rate of platelet recovery, the frequency of infections or the duration of remissions. In two patients, leukemic blasts appeared following commencement of GM-CSF. In one, withdrawal of the growth factor resulted in regression of the blast population. Insufficient patients have been evaluated to assess the risk of leukemic outgrowth with GM-CSF administration. Anecdotal evidence suggests that in some instances cells induced to proliferate by GM-CSF may be growth factor dependent and withdrawal of the CSF can stop proliferation [72].

The use of GM-CSF to induce differentiation of leukemic blast cells in vivo has only been assessed in studies which included cytotoxic-drug administration, and not in studies of patients receiving GM-CSF alone. In early studies performed in patients with myelodysplastic syndromes [14, 73–76], approximately 15%, overall, of reported patients progressed to acute myeloid leukemia (AML). These tended to be patients with more than 10–15% blasts in pretreatment marrow. Given these observations, it appears unlikely that GM-CSF will find widespread utility to prevent or treat leukemic progression by inducing differentiation.

The third approach to leukemic therapy with CSFs is to combine them with chemotherapy in an attempt to increase cytotoxicity. The cytotoxicity of cycle-specific drugs such as cytosine arabinoside depends upon cell cycle status, and up to 10% of leukemic blasts may not cycle during an 8- to 10-day period [77]. In vitro studies have demonstrated that sensitivity to cytosine arabinoside can be increased by the addition of hemopoietic growth factors [78, 79]. IL-3 and GM-CSF have both been shown to increase cytotoxicity, and clinical studies have now been reported which exploit this effect [80–83]. In the first reported study, 18 patients with previously untreated leukemia received standard induction chemotherapy concomitantly with i.v. GM-CSF [80]. GM-CSF administration was started 24–48 h before chemotherapy with the intention of maximizing the proportion of cycling cells. In 4 patients this was not possible because of an initial high white cell count. A complete-response rate of 83% (15/18) was reported with a 3-day reduction in the duration of neutropenia when compared with historical controls. This approach has also been reported in smaller numbers of patients with relapsed or refractory AML [82, 83].

In an Australian study, 15 patients with relapsed or refractory myeloid leukemia received GM-CSF by s.c. injection (5 μg/kg) 72 h before standard induction chemotherapy. GM-CSF was administered during the first 4 days of chemotherapy and then recommended 24 h after chemotherapy ceased. The total white cell count increased in 13/15 patients and in 9 of these the peripheral blast count increased during the 3 days prior to chemotherapy. This was associated with an increase in the thymidine-labelling index of blast cells in the bone marrow as well as Ki67 antigen expression. The complete-response rate was 33% and partial-response rate was 20%. Four induction deaths occurred, three of which were associated with pulmonary leukostasis at relatively low total blast cell counts [unpubl. data, 81].

In another series [82], 56 patients with previously untreated AML received varying doses of GM-CSF for up to 3 days before chemotherapy. The complete-response rate in this group of patients was poorer than in a series of historical controls who received moderately high-dose cytosine arabinoside in combination with an anthracycline. Adjustments were made for a variety of prognostic variables, however the differences between study and control groups makes interpretation difficult.

The true value of GM-CSF in combination with chemotherapy for patients with AML remains unproven and large randomized control studies will be required to establish this.

## Conclusion

GM-CSF may be applied in a variety of ways for the management of patients with a malignant disease. In particular the utility of GM-CSF in marrow and stem cell transplantation is being established by randomized studies. CSF-primed progenitor cell transplants have clearly accelerated time to multilineage myeloid reconstitution and this is likely to have a major impact on autologous transplantation practices. Nonetheless, the role of GM-CSF in such therapies is still evolving. The results of carefully conducted randomized studies must be awaited before the usefulness of GM-CSF in these various applications is defined. These studies are essential to establish the role of GM-CSF in a variety of settings so that its use can be of maximum benefit for patients.

## Acknowledgements

The authors would like to thank Linda Tabone for excellent assistance in preparation of the manuscript and Dr. James Wiley for use of unpublished data. The authors are members of the Melbourne Centre for Developmental Cancer Therapeutics, a Cooperative Centre of the Austin Hospital, Ludwig Institute for Cancer Research, Royal Melbourne Hospital, Walter and Eliza Hall Institute for Medical Research and the Western Hospital, Melbourne, Australia. GJL is supported by the John Maynard Hedstrom Research Fellowship of the Anti-Cancer Council of Victoria.

## References


1 Cebon JS, Morstyn G: The potential of granulocyte-macrophage colony stimulating factor (GM-CSF) in cancer chemotherapy. Cancer Surv 1990;9:131–155.

2 Demetri GD, Antman HS: Granulocyte-macrophage colony-stimulating factor (GM-CSF): Preclinical and clinical investigations. Semin Oncol 1992;19:362–385.

3 Lieschke GJ, Burgees AW: Granulocyte colony stimulating factor and granulocyte macrophage colony stimulating factor. New Engl J Med 1992;327:28–35;99–106.

4 Metcalf D, Morstyn G: Colony stimulating factors: General biology; in De Vita VT Jr, Hellman S, Rosenberg SA (eds): Biologic Therapy of Cancer. Philadelphia, Lippincott, 1991, pp 417–444.

5 Burgess AW, Begley CG, Johnson GR, Lopez AF, Williamson DJ, Mermod JJ, Simpson RJ, Schmitz A, DeLamarter JF: Purification and properties of bacterially synthesized human granulocyte macrophage colony stimulating factor. Blood 1987;69:43–51.

6 Nicola NA, Metcalf D, Matsumoto M, Johnson GR: Purification of a factor inducing differentiation in murine myelomonocytic leukemia cells. Identification as granulocyte colony-stimulating factor. J Biol Chem 1983;258:9017–9023.

7 Demetri GD, Griffin JD: Granulocyte colony stimulating factor and its receptor. Blood 1991;78:2791–2808.

8 Cebon J, Layton J, Pavlovic R, Iaria J, Dyer W, Morstyn G: Endogenous cytokine production in response to sepsis in neutropenic and non-neutropenic patients. Blood 1991;78(suppl): p 8a, abstr 23.

9 Grabstein KH, Urdal DL, Tushinski RJ, Mochizuki DY, Price VL, Cantrell MA, Gillis S, Conlon PJ: Induction of macrophage tumoricidal activity by granulocyte-macrophage colony-stimulating factor. Science 1986;232:506–508.

10 Fischer HG, Frosch S, Reske K, Reske-Kunz AB: Granulocyte-macrophage colony-stimulating factor activates macrophages derived from bone marrow cultures to synthesis of MHC class II molecules and to augmented antigen presentation function. J Immunol 1988;141:3882–3888.

11 Vadas MA, Nicola N, Metcalf D: Activation of antibody-dependent cell-mediated cytotoxicity of human neutrophils and eosinophils by separate colony stimulating factors. J Immunol 1983;130:795–799.

12 Miyauchi J, Kelleher CA, Yang YC, Wong GC, Clark SC, Minden MD, Minkin S, McCulloch EA: The effects of three recombinant growth factors, IL-3, GM-CSF and G-CSF on the blast cells of acute myeloblastic leukemia maintained in short term suspension culture. Blood 1987;70:657–663.

13 Lieschke GJ, Maher D, Cebon J, O'Connor M, Green M, Sheridan W, Boyd A, Rallings M, Bonnem E, Metcalf D, Burgess AW, McGrath K, Fox RM, Morstyn G: Effects of subcutaneously administered bacterially-synthesized recombinant human granulocyte-macrophage colony-stimulating factor in patients with advanced malignancy. Ann Intern Med 1989;110:357–364.

14 Thompson JA, Lee DJ, Kidd P, Rubin E, Kaufmann J, Bonnem EM, Fefer A: Subcutaneous granulocyte macrophage colony stimulating factor in patients with myelodysplastic syndrome: Toxicity, pharmacokinetics, and hematological effects. J Clin Oncol 1989;7:629–637.

15 Ganser A, Völkers B, Greher J, Ottmann OG, Walther F, Becher R, Bergmann L, Schulz G, Hoelzer D: Recombinant human granulocyte-macrophage colony-stimulating factor in patients with myelodysplastic syndromes – a phase I/II trial. Blood 1989;73:31–37.

16 Herrmann F, Schulz G, Lindemann A, Meyenburg W, Oster W, Krumwieh D, Mertelsmann R: Hematopoietic responses in patients with advanced malignancy treated with recombinant human granulocyte-macrophage colony-stimulating factor. J Clin Oncol 1989;7:159–167.

17 Socinski MA, Cannistra SA, Sullivan R, Elias A, Antman K, Schnipper L, Griffin JD: Granulocyte-macrophage colony-stimulating factor induces the expression of CD11b surface adhesion molecule on human granulocytes in vivo. Blood 1988;72:691–697.

18 Devereux S, Bull HA, Campos-Costa D, Saib R, Linch DC: Granulocyte macrophage colony stimulating factor induced changes in cellular adhesion molecule expression and adhesion to endothelium: In vitro and in vivo studies in man. Br J Haematol 1989;71:323–330.

19 Sullivan R, Fredette JP, Socinski M, Elias A, Antman K, Schnipper L, Griffin JD: Enhancement of superoxide anion release by granulocytes harvested from patients receiving granulocyte-macrophage colony-stimulating factor. Br J Haematol 1989;71:475–479.

20 Buescher SE, McIlheran SM, Vadhan-Raj S: Effects of in vivo administration of recombinant human granulocyte-macrophage colony-stimulating factor on human neutrophil chemotaxis and oxygen metabolism. J Infect Dis 1988;158:1140.

21 Antman K, Griffin J, Elias A, Socinski MA, Ryan L, Cannistra SA, Oette D, Whitley M, Frei E III, Schnipper LE: Effect of recombinant human granulocyte-macrophage colony stimulating factor on chemotherapy-induced myelosuppression. N Engl J Med 1988;319:593–598.

22 Herrmann F, Schulz G, Wiesier M, Kolbe K, Nicolay U, Noack M, Lindemann A, Mertelsmann R: Effect of granulocyte-macrophage colony-stimulating factor on neutropenia and related morbidity induced by myelotoxic chemotherapy. Am J Med 1990;88:619–624.

23 de Vries EGE, Biesma B, Willemse PHB, Mulder NH, Stern AC, Aalders JG, Vellenga E: A double-blind placebo-controlled study with granulocyte-macrophage colony stimulating factor during chemotherapy for ovarian carcinoma. Cancer Res 1991;51:116–122.

24 Edmonson JH, Colon-Otero G, Long HJ, Fitch TR, Jeffries JA, Buckner JC, Rubin J, Braich TA: Granulocyte-macrophage colony-stimulating factor (GM-CSF) permits escalation of carboplatin (CBDCA) doses (abstract 330). Proc Am Soc Clin Oncol 1990;9:85.

25 Lichtman S, Ratain M, Budman DR, Norton L, Egorin M, Propert K, Modeas C, Paterson D, Van Echo DA: Phase I trial of recombinant granulocyte-macrophage colony stimulating factor (GM-CSF) plus cyclophosphamide (CYC) in solid tumors. Blood 1989;74(suppl): 328.

26 Bishop JF, Morstyn G, Stuart-Harris R, Green M, Matthews J, Zalcberg J, Kefford R, Yuen K, Ball D, Olver I, Cebon J, Raghavan D, Zimet A, Fox R: The dose and schedule of granulocyte macrophage colony stimulating factor (GM-CSF) carboplatin and etoposide in small cell lung cancer, submitted.

27 Vadhan-Raj S, Broxmeyer HE, Hittelman WN, Papadopoulos NE, Chawla SP, Fenoglio C, Cooper S, Buescher ES, Frenck RW Jr, Holian A, Perkins RC, Scheule RK, Gutterman JU, Salem P, Benjamin RS: Abrogating chemotherapy-induced myelosuppression by recombinant granulocyte-macrophage colony-stimulating factor in patients with sarcoma: Protection at the progenitor cell level. J Clin Oncol 1992;10:1266–1277.

28 Gianni A, Bregni M, Siena S, Orazi A, Stern AC, Gandola L, Bonadonna G: Recombinant human granulocyte-macrophage colony-stimulating factor reduces hematologic toxicity and widens clinical applicability of high-dose cyclophosphamide treatment in breast cancer and non-Hodgkin's lymphoma. J Clin Oncol 1990;8:768–778.

29 Bronchud MH, Howell A, Crowther D, Hopwood P, Souza L, Dexter TM: The use of granulocyte colony-stimulating factor to increase the intensity of treatment with doxorubicin in patients with advanced breast and ovarian cancer. Br J Cancer 1989;60:121–125.

30 Hoekman K, Wagstaff J, van-Groeningen CJ, Vermorken JB, Boven E, Pinedo HM: Effects of recombinant human granulocyte-macrophage colony-stimulating factor on myelosuppression induced by multiple cycles of high-dose chemotherapy in patients with advanced breast cancer. J Natl Cancer Inst 1991;83:1546–1553.

31 Shea TC, Mason JR, Newton B, Storniolo AM, Taetle R, Green MR: High-dose carboplatin (CBDCA) with recombinant human granulocyte-macrophage colony stimulating factor (rHu-GM-CSF): A phase I study (abstract 1109). Proc Am Soc Clin Oncol 1990;9:286.

32 Barlogie B, Jagannath S, Dixon DO, Cheson B, Smallwood L, Hendrickson A, Purvis JD, Bonnem E, Alexanian R: High-dose melphalan and granulocyte-macrophage colony-stimulating factor for refractory multiple myeloma. Blood 1990;76:677–680.

33 O'Dwyer PJ, LaCreta FP, Schilder R, Nash S, McAleer C, Miller LL, Hudes GR, Ozols RF: Phase I trial of thiotepa in combination with recombinant human granulocyte-macrophage colony-stimulating factor. J Clin Oncol 1992; 10:1352–1358.

34 Gurney H, Anderson H, Radford J, Potter MR, Swindell R, Steward W, Kamthan A, Chang J, Weiner J, Thatcher N, Crowther D: Infection risk in patients with small cell lung cancer receiving intensive chemotherapy and recombinant human granulocyte-macrophage colony-stimulating factor. Eur J Cancer 1992;28: 105–112.

35 Steward WP, Scarffe JH, Dirix LY, Chang J, Radford JA, Bonnem E, Crowther D: Granulocyte-macrophage colony-stimulating factor (GM-CSF) after high-dose melphalan in patients with advanced colon cancer. Br J Cancer 1990;61:749–754.

36 Neidhart J, Stidley C, Ferguson J, Mangalik A, Anderson T, Oldham F: GM-CSF decreases duration of cytopenia in patients receiving dose intensive therapy with cyclophosphamide (C), etoposide (E), and cisplatin (P) (abstract 753). Proc Am Soc Clin Oncol 1990;9:195.

37 Logothetis CJ, Dexeus FH, Sella A, Amato RJ, Kilbourn RG, Finn L, Gutterman JU: Escalated therapy for refractory urethelial tumors: Methotrexate-vinblastine-doxorubicin-cisplatin plus unglycosylated recombinant human granulocyte-macrophage colony-stimulating factor. J Natl Cancer Inst 1990;82:667–672.

38 Ho AD, Del Valle F, Engelhard M, Hiddemann W, Ruckle H, Schlimok G, Haas R, Thiel E, Andreesen R, Fiedler W, Frisch J, Schulz G, Hunstein W: Mitoxantrone/high-dose Ara-C and recombinant human GM-CSF in the treatment of refractory non-Hodgkin's lymphoma. A pilot study. Cancer 1990;66:423–430.

39 Kantarjian HM, Estey EH, O'Brien S, Anaissie E, Beran M, Rios MB, Keating MJ, Gutterman MJ: Intensive chemotherapy with mitoxantrone and high-dose cytosine arabinoside followed by granulocyte-macrophage colony-stimulating factor in the treatment of patients with acute lymphocytic leukemia. Blood 1992;79: 876–881.

40 Gerhartz HH, Engelhard M, Brittinger G, Wilmanns W, Huhn D, Thiel E, Huber C, Schlimok G, Gerhartz D, Emmerich B, Kabelitz K, Schadek D, Pees HW, Deupmann F, Schick H, Schaefer M, Brandmeier R, Hasford S, Stern AC, Jones T: Randomized double-blind placebo-controlled phase III study of recombinant human granulocyte/macrophage colony stimulating factor (rhGM-CSF) in patients treated for non-Hodgkin's lymphomas. Blood 1992; 80(suppl 1):78a.

41 Schulz G, Frisch J, Greifenberg B, Nicolay U, Oster W: New therapeutic modalities for the clinical use of rhGM-CSF in patients with malignancies. Am J Clin Oncol 1991;14(suppl 1): S19–26.

42 Rusthoven J, Levin L, Eisenhauer E, Mazurka J, Carmichael J, O'Connell G, Bryson P, Hirte H, Koski B: Two phase I studies of carboplatin dose escalation in chemotherapy-naive ovarian cancer patients supported with granulocyte-macrophage colony-stimulating factor. J Natl Cancer Inst 1991;83:1748–1753.

43 Neidhart JA: Hematopoietic colony-stimulating factors. Use in combination with standard chemotherapeutic regimens and in support of dose intensification. Cancer Suppl 1992;70: 913–920.

44 Edmonson JH, Long HJ, Jeffries JA: Amelioration of chemotherapy-induced thrombocytopenia by GM-CSF: Apparent dose and schedule dependency. J Natl Cancer Inst 1989;81:1510–1512.

45 Brandt SJ, Peters WP, Atwater SK, Kurtzberg J, Borowitz MJ, Jones RB, Shpall EJ, Bast RC, Gilbert CJ, Oette DH: Effect of recombinant human granulocyte-macrophage colony-stimulating factor on hematopoietic reconstitution after high-dose chemotherapy and autologous bone marrow transplantation. New Engl J Med 1988;318:869–876.

46 Nemunaitis J, Singer JW, Buckner CD, Hill R, Storb R, Thomas ED, Appelbau FR: Use of recombinant human granulocyte-macrophage colony-stimulating factor in autologous marrow transplantation for lymphoid malignancies. Blood 1988;72:834–836.

47 Blazar BR, Kersev JH, McGlave PB, Vallera DA, Lasky LC, Haake RJ, Bostrom B, Weisdorf DR, Epstein C, Ramsay NKC: In vivo administration of recombinant human granulocyte macrophage colony-stimulating factor in acute lymphoblastic leukemia patients receiving purged autografts. Blood 1989;73:849–857.

48 Devereux S, Linch DC, Gribben JG, McMillan A, Patterson K, Goldstone AH: GM-CSF accelerates neutrophil recovery after autologous bone marrow transplantation for Hodgkin's disease. Bone Marrow Transplant 1989;4:49–54.

49 Nemunaitis JN, Rabinowe SN, Singer JW, Bierman PH, Vose JM, Freedman AS, Onetto N, Gillis S, Oette D, Gold M, Buckner CD, Hansen JA, Ritz J, Appelbaum FR, Armitage JO, Nadler LM: Recombinant granulocyte-macrophage colony-stimulating factor after autologous bone marrow transplantation for lymphoid cancer. N Engl J Med 1991;324:1773–1778.

50 Advani R, Chao NJ, Horning SJ, Blume KG, Ahn DK, Lamborn KR, Fleming NC, Bonnem EM, Greenberg PL: Granulocyte-macrophage colony-stimulating factor (GM-CSF) as an adjunct to autologous hemopoietic stem cell transplantation for lymphoma. Ann Intern Med 1992;116:183–189.

51 Gulati SC, Bennett CL: Granulocyte-macrophage colony-stimulating factor (GM-CSF) as adjunct therapy in relapsed Hodgkin disease. Ann Intern Med 1992;116:177–182.

52 Khwaja A, Linch DC, Goldstone AH, Chopra R, Marcus RE, Wimperis JZ, Russell NH, Haynes AP, Milligan DW, Leyland MJ, Winfield DA, Hancock BW, Newland A, Durrant ST, Devereux S, Roitt S, Collins M, Hudson GV: Recombinant human granulocyte-macrophage colony-stimulating factor after autologous bone marrow transplantation for malignant lymphoma: A British national lymphoma investigation double-blind, placebo-controlled trial. Br J Haematol 1992;82:317–323.

53 Gorin NC, Coiffier B, Hayat M, Fouillard L, Kuentz M, Flesch M, Colombat P, Boivin P, Slavin S, Philip T: Recombinant human granulocyte-macrophage colony-stimulating factor after high dose chemotherapy and autologous bone marrow transplantation with unpurged marrow in non-Hodgkin's lymphoma: A double blind placebo-controlled trial. Blood 1992; 80:1149–1157.

54 Link H, Boogaerts M, Carella A, Ferrant A, Gadner H, Gorin NC, Harabacz I, Harrousseau F, Herve P, Kolb HJ, Krieger O, Labar B, Linkesch W, Mandelli F, Maranchini D, Nicolay U, Niederwieser D, Reiffers J, Rizzoli V, Siegert W, Slavin S, Vernant JP, de Witte T: Recombinant human granulocyte-macrophage colony stimulating factor after autologous bone marrow transplantation for acute lymphoblastic leukemia and non-Hodgkin's lymphoma: A randomized double blind multicenter trial in Europa (abstract). Blood 1990;76:152a.

55 Nemunaitis J, Buckner CJ, Appelbaum FR, Higano CS, Mor M, Bianco J, Epstein C, Lipani J, Hansen J, Storb R, Thomas ED, Singer JW: Phase I/II trial of recombinant human granulocyte-macrophage colony-stimulating factor following allogeneic bone marrow transplantation. Blood 1991;77:2065–2071.

56 De Witte T, Gratwohl A, Van Der Lely N, Bacigalupo A, Stern AC, Speck B, Schattenberg A, Nissen C, Gluckman E, Fibbe WE: Recombinant human granulocyte-macrophage colony-stimulating factor accelerates neutrophil and monocyte recovery after allogeneic T-cell-depleted bone marrow transplantation. Blood 1992;79:1359–1365.

57 Powles R, Smith C, Milan S, Treleaven J, Millar J, McElwain T, Gordon-Smith E, Milliken S, Tiley C: Human recombinant GM-CSF in allogeneic bone-marrow transplantation for leukaemia: Double blind, placebo controlled trial. Lancet 1990;336:1417–1420.

58 Richman CM, Weuner RS, Yankee RA: Increase in circulating stem cells following chemotherapy in man. Blood 1976;47:1031–1039.

59 Socinski MA, Cannistra SA, Elias A, Antman KH, Schnipper L, Griffin JD: Granulocyte-macrophage colony stimulating factor expands the circulating haemopoietic progenitor cell compartment in man. Lancet 1988;1:1194–1198.

60 Villeval JL, Dührsen U, Morstyn G, Metcalf D: Effect of recombinant human granulocyte-macrophage colony stimulating factor on hemopoietic progenitor cells in patients with advanced malignancies. Br J Haematol 1990;74:36.

61 Dührsen U, Villeval JL, Boyd J, Kannourakis G, Morstyn G, Metcalf D: Effects of recombinant human granulocyte colony stimulating factor on haemopoietic progenitor cells in cancer patients. Blood 1988;72:2074–2081.

62 To LB, Dyson PG, Bradford A: Peripheral blood stem cells collected in very early remission produce rapid and sustained autologous hemopoietic reconstitution in acute non-lymphoblastic leukemia. Bone Marrow Transplant 1987;2:103–108.

63 Gianni AM, Siena S, Bregni M, Tarella C, Stern AC, Pileri A, Bonadonna G: Granulocyte-macrophage colony-stimulating factor to harvest circulating haemopoietic stem cells for autotransplantation. Lancet 1989;ii:580–585.

64 Elias AD, Ayashi L, Anderson KC, Hunt M, Wheeler C, Schwartz G, Tepler I, Mazanet R, Lynch C, Pap S, Pelaez J, Reich E, Critchlow J, Demetri G, Bibbo J, Schnipper L, Griffin JD, Frei E III, Antman KH: Mobilization of peripheral blood progenitor cells by chemotherapy and granulocyte-macrophage colony-stimulating factor for hematologic support after high-dose intensification for breast cancer. Blood 1992;79:3036–3044.

65 Korbling M, Holle R, Haas R, Knauf W, Dorken B, Ho AD, Kuse R, Pralle H, Fliedner TM, Hunstein W: Autologous blood stem-cell transplantation in patients with advanced Hodgkin's disease and prior radiation to the pelvic site. J Clin Oncol 1990;8:978–985.

66 Haas R, Ho AD, Bredthauer U, Cayeux S, Egerer G, Knauf W, Hunstein W: Successful autologous transplantation of blood stem cells mobilized with recombinant human granulocyte-macrophage colony-stimulating factor. Exp Hematol 1990;18:94–98.

67 Brugger W, Bross K, Frisch J, Dern P, Weber B, Mertelsmann R, Kanz L: Mobilization of peripheral blood progenitor cells by sequential administration of interleukin-3 and granulocyte-macrophage colony-stimulating factor following polychemotherapy with etoposide, ifosfamide, and cisplatin. Blood 1992;79:1193–1200.

68 Mazanet R, Elias A, Hunt M, Ayash L, Anderson K, Wheeler C, Schwartz G, Tepler I, Critchlow J, Schnipper L, Demetri G, Griffin J, Frei E III, Antman K: Peripheral blood progenitor cells (PBPC)s added to bone marrow (BM) for hemopoietic rescue following high dose chemotherapy for solid tumors reduces morbidity and length of hospitalization (abstract 1140). Proc Am Soc Clin Oncol 1991;10:324.

69 Sheridan WP, Begley CG, Juttner CA, Szer J, To LB, Maher D, McGrath KM, Morstyn G, Fox RM: Effect of peripheral-blood progenitor cells mobilised by filgrastim (G-CSF) on platelet recovery after high-dose chemotherapy. Lancet 1992;339:640–644.

70 Ravagnani F, Siena S, Bregni M, Sciorelli G, Gianni AM, Pellegris G: Large-scale collection of circulating haematopoietic progenitors in cancer patients treated with high-dose cyclophosphamide and recombinant human GM-CSF. Eur J Cancer 1990;26:562–564.

71 Lieschke GJ, Ramenghi U, O'Connor MP, Sheridan W, Szer J: Studies of oral neutrophil levels in patients receiving G-CSF after autologous marrow transplantation. Br J Hematol 1992;82:589–595.

72 Buchner T, Hiddemann W, Koenigsmann M, Zühlsdorf M, Wörmann B, Boeckmann A, Freire EA, Innig C, Maschmeyer G, Ludwig WD, Sauerland MC, Heinecke A, Schulz G: Recombinant human granulocyte-macrophage colony-stimulating factor after chemotherapy in patients with acute myeloid leukemia at higher age of after relapse. Blood 1991;78:1190–1197.

73 Vadhan-Raj S, Keating M, LeMaistre A, Hittelman WN, McCredie K, Trujillo JM, Broxmeyer HE, Henney C, Gutterman JU: Effects of recombinant human granulocyte-macrophage colony-stimulating factor in patients with myelodysplastic syndromes. N Engl J Med 1987;317:1545–1552.

74 Antin JH, Weinberg DS, Rosenthal DS: Variable effect of recombinant human granulocyte-macrophage colony-stimulating factor on bone marrow fibrosis in patients with myelodysplasia. Exp Hematol 1990;18:266–270.

75 Ganser A, Volkers B, Greher J, Ottmann OG, Walther F, Becher R, Bergmann L, Schulz G, Hoelzer D: Recombinant human granulocyte-macrophage colony-stimulating factor in patients with myelodysplastic syndromes – a phase I/II trial. Blood 1989;73:31–37.

76 Herrmann F, Lindemann A, Klein H, Lubbert M, Schulz G, Mertelsmann R: Effect of recombinant human granulocyte macrophage colony stimulating factor in patients with myelodysplastic syndrome with excess blasts. Leukemia 1989;3:335–338.

77 Clarkson B, Strife A, Fried J, Sakai Y, Ota K, Ohkita T, Masuda R: Studies of cellular proliferation in human leukemia IV. Behaviour of leukemic cells in 3 adults with acute leukemia given continuous infusions of 3H-thymidine for 8–10 days. Cancer 1970;26:1–19.

78 Cannistra SA, Groshek P, Griffin JD: Granulocyte macrophage colony-stimulating factor enhances the cytotoxic effects of cytosine arabinoside in acute myeloblastic leukemia and in the myeloid blast crisis phase of chronic myeloid leukemia. Leukemia 1989;3:328–334.

79 Bhalla K, Birkhofer M, Arlin Z, Grant S, Lutzky J, Graham G: Effect of recombinant GM-CSF on the metabolism of cytosine arabinoside in normal and leukemic human bone marrow cells. Leukemia 1988;2:810–813.

80 Bettelheim P, Valent P, Andreeff M, Tafuri A, Haimi J, Gorischek C, Muhm M, Sillaber CH, Haas O, Vieder L, Mauer D, Schulz G, Speiser W, Geissler K, Kier P, Hinterberger W, Lechner K: Recombinant human granulocyte-macrophage colony-stimulating factor in combination with standard induction chemotherapy in de novo acute myeloid leukemia. Blood 1991;77:700–711.

81 Wiley J, Cebon J, Woodruff R, Jamieson G, Snook M, McKendrick J, Szer J, Dennington P, Sheridan W, Begley G, van der Weyden M, Fox R: Granulocyte-macrophage colony stimulating factor followed by chemotherapy in the treatment of poor prognosis acute myeloid leukemia. Blood 1991;78(suppl):42a.

82 Estey E, Thall PF, Kantarjian H, O'Brien S, Koller CA, Beran M, Gutterman J, Deisseroth A, Keating M: Treatment of newly diagnosed acute myelogenous leukemia with granulocyte-macrophage colony-stimulating factor (GM-CSF) before and during continuous-infusion high-dose ara-C + daunorubicin: Comparison to patients treated without GM-CSF. Blood 1992;79:2246–2255.

83 Cannistra SA, DiCarlo J, Groshek P, Kanakura Y, Berg D, Mayer RJ, Griffin JD: Simultaneous administration of granulocyte-macrophage colony-stimulating factor and cytosine arabinoside for the treatment of relapsed acute myeloid leukemia. Leukemia 1991;5:230–238.

Oncology 1994;51:189–197

*M.H. Bronchud*

Developmental Therapeutics Unit,
Department of Hematology,
Hospital of San Pablo, Barcelona, Spain

# Recombinant Human Granulocyte Colony-Stimulating Factor in the Management of Cancer Patients: Five Years On

**Key Words**
Granulocyte colony-stimulating-factor
Cancer chemotherapy
Febrile neutropenia
Dose intensity

**Abstract**
Recombinant human granulocyte colony-stimulating factor (G-CSF) has been used worldwide in cancer patients for over 1 year, and (only 5 years from the first publication on the clinical use of this growth factor) experience is rapidly accumulating in many oncological situations. Several randomized studies have confirmed its value in allowing the optimal delivery of chemotherapy without undue dose reductions or dose delays, while at the same time reducing the overall risks of febrile neutropenia associated with the use of cytotoxic chemotherapy. Its virtual lack of significant side effects, its selectivity of action, its rapid effect on neutrophil kinetics (reducing both the maturation and release times of bone marrow neutrophils to 1–2 days rather than the normal 4–5 days), and the reproducible augmentation of neutrophil production in several neoplastic and nonneoplastic situations, as well as the activation of myeloid cell functions, have made G-CSF the growth factor of choice in most cancer units. Some of the published information regarding its current and potential use in the management of oncological patients is summarized here.

## Introduction

Cytotoxic drugs used at curative doses produce a variety of side effects which range in severity from mild to life-threatening. Combinations of drugs tend to include drugs with nonoverlapping toxicities, which helps to avoid additive damage to a particular organ, but increases the range of adverse effects experienced. The major dose-limiting toxicity for many combination regimens is myelosuppression.

Bone marrow toxicity leads to the development of neutropenia and thrombocytopenia which increase the risk of infection and requirements for platelet transfusions, respectively. The risk of infection is closely related to the degree and duration of neutropenia [1]. Neutropenic infection requires hospitalization and immediate treatment with broad-spectrum intravenous antibiotics. Despite such treatment, morbidity is significant and the mortality rate may be as high as 5–20%. The most serious consequence of neutropenia and infection, however, may

Dr. M.H. Bronchud
Developmental Therapeutics Unit
Department of Hematology, Hospital of San Pablo
Antonio M. Claret 167
E–08025 Barcelona (Spain)


0030–2414/94/0512–0189
$5.00/0

be dose reduction or delay, leading to a decrease in chemotherapy dose intensity and an adverse effect on treatment outcome [2]. Furthermore, myelosuppression limits attempts to further increase doses in an attempt to improve treatment outcome in poor-risk patients.

The introduction of hematopoietic growth factors offers clinicians the opportunity to reduce the impact of neutropenia on treatment strategies and thus may lead to an enhanced ability to deliver regimens as planned without the need for dose modification as a result of myelotoxicity. The hematopoietic growth factors play a fundamental role in regulating the production of at least eight different types of mature cells found in peripheral blood. Evidence of their biological activity has been demonstrated for over two decades, but only recently has recombinant DNA technology enabled the production of sufficient amounts of these factors for clinical use. Four myeloid hematopoietic growth factors have been isolated in mouse and humans which differ in their proliferative potential for the granulocyte-macrophage populations [3]. Two have a relatively restricted proliferative effect: granulocyte colony-stimulating factor (G-CSF) predominantly stimulates neutrophil granulocyte formation, while macrophage colony-stimulating factor (M-CSF) stimulates the formation of monocytes and macrophages. Interleukin-3 (IL-3) and granulocyte-macrophage colony stimulating factor (GM-CSF) are less specific and stimulate the formation of both cell types, although at a low concentration GM-CSF tends to stimulate only the proliferation of monocytes and macrophages. The results of early clinical studies using G-CSF, GM-CSF, M-CSF and IL-3 in humans have been reported [4] and some are summarized in other chapters of this supplement.

The immediate effect of G-CSF and GM-CSF is a transient fall in the white blood cell (WBC) count, occurring minutes after bolus injection. This is followed 6–12 h later, with G-CSF, by an increase in neutrophil counts. The increase in the WBC count following GM-CSF is less rapid and involves a broader range of cells. The early effects, occurring within 24 h, may be attributable to an accelerated release from a preformed pool of granulocytes in bone marrow, to demargination from endothelial adherent pools, and to prolonged survival in the circulation. With continued administration, there is a dose-dependent increase in WBCs, although there are individual variations, up to very high levels, with the appearance of immature precursors in peripheral blood [5]. When G-CSF is administered, the increase in WBCs is mainly caused by a rise in neutrophils. The principal cause of an increased WBC count after GM-CSF treatment is also neutrophilia, although eosinophils and monocytes also increase. Both growth factors increase the neutrophil count through amplification in the bone marrow maturation compartment. With G-CSF, newly formed neutrophils are released after a very short time compared to the normal situation 1 day versus 5 [6, 7].

### Effects of G-CSF after Conventional Chemotherapy

Both G-CSF and GM-CSF have demonstrated clinical benefits in studies involving cancer patients receiving chemotherapy for a variety of malignancies [8, 9]. For example, those studies which have directly compared cycles of chemotherapy with or without recombinant human (rh) G-CSF have reported a reduction in the number of febrile days, a reduced incidence of infections and, as a result, fewer days on antibiotics [10–16]. A shorter duration of neutropenia was seen in patients receiving G-CSF, independent of whether it was administered in the first or second treatment cycle. An additional benefit may be a reduction in the degree of mucositis experienced by patients [12].

Two randomized, double-blind, phase III trials involving 314 patients with small cell lung cancer receiving intensive chemotherapy demonstrated that G-CSF significantly reduced the incidence of febrile neutropenia compared with placebo [15, 16]. The risk of being hospitalized for infection, and the total duration of hospitalization were also significantly reduced by G-CSF compared with placebo on the first cycle of chemotherapy. The benefits of G-CSF were maintained over all six cycles of chemotherapy. The conclusions from preclinical and clinical studies are summarized below.

G-CSF is well-tolerated when administered by either the subcutaneous or intravenous routes. Very few side effects were reported for rhG-CSF during phase I-III studies. Like GM-CSF, it is associated with dose-dependent and manageable musculoskeletal pains, but, unlike GM-CSF, it is not associated with fever, malaise, anorexia, chills or more severe toxicities, and no clear maximum tolerated dose has been described for G-CSF. The musculoskeletal pains affecting some 8–18% of patients (localizing mainly at the sternum, pelvis, limbs and back) are frequently described as a dull ache and are usually relieved by paracetamol. Like GM-CSF, G-CSF can induce raised levels of serum lactate dehydrogenase and alkaline phosphatase (probably of leukocyte or bony origins) and, less frequently, mild alterations of liver transaminases and bilirubin have also been reported [17].

G-CSF does not appear to require the input of earlier pluripotent cells, and there seems to be no experimental or clinical evidence of exhaustion of the human hematopoietic system if the treatments are repeated [6]. However, when stem cell function was recently assessed by serially transferred bone marrow cells from high-dose-cyclophosphamide- and CSF- (either G-CSF or GM-CSF) treated mice into lethally irradiated recipient mice, it was found that bone marrow cells from animals treated with CSFs lost more rapidly the ability to repopulate the recipient lymphoid organs and, following the third consecutive serial transplant, experienced a 40–50% reduction in marrow repopulating ability [18]. In an accompanying editorial, Moore [19] reminds us that preclinical models in mice and monkeys demonstrated that continuous administration of CSFs, during or very shortly before or after chemotherapy, could be counterproductive; so it seemed necessary to build in certain 'wash-out' periods before and after each chemotherapy cycle. The same author ironically comments that determining the duration of such 'wash-outs' has been less than an exact science and more studies should be encouraged to answer this question. G-CSF administered postchemotherapy usually leads to a decrease in the time interval between day 1 after chemotherapy and the onset of nadir neutropenia (T1), but because it also leads to a marked acceleration in the recovery time from nadir (T2: time interval between day 1 after chemotherapy and a return to normal peripheral neutrophil counts), G-CSF substantially reduces the overall period of severe neutropenia (probably by about 50% in most studies). The actual mechanisms responsible for these two kinetic effects are probably quite different, at both cellular and molecular levels, and need to be studied further [22].

Neutrophils produced following stimulation with G-CSF are functionally normal [20, 21]. This also appears to be the case with GM-CSF, although one trial reported a deficit in neutrophil migration [23].

Although some studies have demonstrated the presence of hematopoietic growth factor receptors on tumor cells [24], there is no clinical evidence of enhancement of nonmyeloid tumor cell growth in vivo with G-CSF. Preliminary reports on the clinical use of G-CSF in myeloid malignancies [25] do not confirm a stimulatory effect on leukemia recurrence or a negative effect on overall survival, but should be followed by larger prospective randomized trials.

Two randomized, double-blind, placebo-controlled trials (n = 314) have shown that G-CSF reduces the incidence of febrile neutropenia (by about 50%) and the duration of neutropenia [15, 16]. This is associated with reduced total days of hospitalization for infection, a decreased requirement for intravenous antibiotics and an improved ability to deliver chemotherapy on schedule.

Clinical trials have clearly shown that G-CSF facilitates the delivery of cytotoxic chemotherapy. Clear evidence for this effect was provided by the European randomized, double-blind, placebo-controlled trial in 130 patients with small cell lung cancer [16]. Patients received CDE chemotherapy followed by G-CSF or placebo for six cycles. The same rules for dose modification were applied to both treatment groups. Treatment was delayed for 7 days if the absolute neutrophil count (ANC) was $<2.0 \times 10^9/l$ or platelets were $<100 \times 10^9/l$; a 25% dose reduction was made if the patient experienced febrile neutropenia or WHO grade IV toxicity; a 50% dose reduction was made for ANC $<1.0 \times 10^9/l$ or platelets $<20 \times 10^9/l$ for 6 or more days, or consecutive WHO grade IV toxicity. The trial showed that G-CSF significantly reduced both the need to delay administration and the need to reduce the dose of chemotherapy. Patients on placebo were 1.6-fold more likely to suffer a treatment delay of 2 or more days and 2.0-fold more likely to have their dose of chemotherapy reduced by 25% or more, compared with patients on G-CSF. As a result of the reduced need to dose-modify, patients in the G-CSF group received a higher cumulative dose and a greater chemotherapy dose intensity [16]. Both the American and European trials [15, 16], however, were not designed to detect whether a higher dose intensity had an effect on treatment outcome.

Further data showing that G-CSF facilitates chemotherapy delivery were provided by a phase II trial in patients with bladder cancer receiving M-VAC. Day 14 chemotherapy is considered part of the optimum administration of M-VAC in bladder cancer and one of the main objectives of this study was to determine whether patients could achieve sufficient neutrophil recovery after M-VAC to enable retreatment 14 days later. During cycles of M-VAC given with G-CSF, all 18 patients achieved an absolute granulocyte count $\geq 2 \times 10^9/l$ on day 14 of the cycle. In contrast, only 5 of 17 patients achieved neutrophil recovery by day 14 during cycles of M-VAC given without G-CSF ($p = 0.001$) [12]. In this same study, patients treated with G-CSF appeared to suffer less severe mucositis than patients not treated with the growth factor. Patients are particular at risk of mucositis and infection in the oral cavity during the neutropenic period after chemotherapy. A recent study of oral neutrophil levels (measured conventionally in routine mouth-rinses) in patients receiving G-CSF after autologous bone marrow transplantation (ABMT) has confirmed that patients treated with G-CSF experience less mucositis and an earlier recovery in oral neutrophil numbers [26].

Both Hodgkin's disease and non-Hodgkin's lymphomas (NHL) are prototypes of chemosensitive malignancies curable by chemotherapy alone and are therefore good models to study dose intensity. The use of rhG-CSF has been shown to reduce myelosuppression and neutropenic fever, and to allow the administration of chemotherapy on schedule both for conventional CHOP-type chemotherapies [27] and for intensive weekly chemotherapies [28]. The Christie hospital group, in England, have recently described a randomized trial of rhG-CSF to preserve the dose-intensity of a new weekly regimen (VAPEC-B, which substitutes methotrexate for VP-16 in a MACOP-B-type protocol) in NHL [28]. Again, as with the multicenter randomized phase III studies in small cell lung cancer, the prophylactic use of rhG-CSF reduced severe neutropenia and neutropenic fever by about 50%, and allowed the administration of chemotherapy on schedule without dose reduction in over 90% of patients. This resulted in slightly more thrombocytopenia and anemia not complicated by clinical sequelae. As in a previous study with adriamycin administered at high dose and dose rates [29], mucositis (and not severe neutropenia) became dose-limiting in some patients. Several European and American groups have gone a stage further and are now investigating the early use of high-dose consolidation therapy with CSF and circulating progenitor cells in subsets of patients with high-grade NHL at high risk of relapse during first remission. In a more conservative, but equally interesting, approach, several groups are experimenting with CHOP given twice weekly (rather than the conventional three times per week) with the help of rhG-CSF. Because of its rapid stimulation of neutrophil kinetics, rhG-CSF is ideally suited for this type of semiweekly myelosuppressive therapy [6]. Steinke et al. [30] have recently reported a study in which 24 patients with high-grade NHL were treated with VIM/CHOP chemotherapy (alternating) at reduced intervals (down to twice weekly): it was possible to apply chemotherapy in the scheduled reduced interval in more than 80% of the cycles without major complications. The complete response (CR) rate was 33%, and the overall response rate 70%.

Thus, although the weight of clinical evidence, albeit retrospective, demonstrates that dose intensity is an important factor determining treatment outcome in lymphoma, and that excessive dose reduction or treatment delay is one of the most important reasons for failure to cure in NHL, we can accept that 'less chemotherapy is worse', but we remain unsure as to whether 'more chemotherapy' is necessarily better [31, 32]. Randomized trials are required to determine whether improved chemotherapy delivery made possible with G-CSF leads to a better treatment outcome.

Patients with refractory or recurrent lymphoma present several clinical problems and their therapy (which cannot yet be said to provide significant, more than 50%, and reproducible CR rates) should ideally remain linked to research protocols in an attempt to get valid and non-anecdotal answers. In this population of patients, the prophylactic use of hemopoietic growth factors can be of particular help, considering that many of these patients have had extensive chemotherapy and, in some cases, also radiotherapy, leading to poor marrow function or decreased hemopoietic recovery. Moreover, bone marrow infiltration by lymphoma is not uncommon in these patients and they seldom tolerate conventional doses of cytotoxic drugs. On the other hand, these patients should be treated with maximum drug doses, in the hope that the apparently drug-resistant clones of tumor cells might become sensitive to higher doses (the concept of 'relative drug resistance'). This latter phenomenon, although infrequent, is probably seen more often in patients with Hodgkin's disease than NHL. Lymphomas in the elderly and in patients with AIDS pose similarly difficult problems, since their hemopoietic tolerance to chemotherapy is poor and dose intensification more often proves counterproductive because of iatrogenic complications and deaths. The prophylactic use of G-CSF in these patient populations could lead to a better tolerance of the conventional nonintensive chemotherapy protocols, and several current studies are addressing these issues.

Histopathological features and the natural history of lymphomas in adults are not the same as for lymphomas in childhood. Marrow and cerebrospinal fluid involvement in children are not infrequently seen in both T and B cell NHL. In the case of B cell disease, heavy infiltration of the bone marrow is usually classified as leukemia and is characteristically associated with a high incidence of testicular and CNS involvement. Chemotherapy treatments need to be intensive to eradicate the disease, and the same is true for other childhood cancers including acute lymphocytic leukemias and neuroblastomas. Recombinant human CSFs are now being investigated in children [33, 34] and are widely used in pediatric clinics with very good responses. These factors may contribute to a better hematological tolerance of chemotherapy in children than in adults, and may be part of the reason why children are more often cured, even in the presence of disseminated disease. It is therefore no surprise that CSFs are also successful in the management of children with lymphomas, both added to conventional protocols and in conjunction with intensive high-dose therapies with circulating progenitor cell support [35].

Combined radiotherapy-chemotherapy is commonly employed for stage I/II NHL and increasingly used also for Hodgkin's disease. It is also indicated as consolidation in areas of previous bulky disease postcytoreduction with chemotherapy in lymphomas, and as an aid to achieve local control in a variety of solid tumors. One of the difficulties with this type of combined modality treatment is the myelosuppression which can lead to dose delays or dose reductions. Although no clinical studies have yet been fully published on the use of CSFs in this setting, it is encouraging that several preliminary reports (including a Japanese randomized and double-blind controlled study) suggest that the administration of rhG-CSF to patients receiving radiotherapy has a definite and reproducible bone marrow protective effect [36]. However, the dose and timing of rhG-CSF administration in relation to the fractionation and timing of radiotherapy need to be better defined.

### High-Dose Chemotherapy and G-CSF

A dose-response relationship for chemosensitive malignancies is evident in experimental models [37] and in retrospective analyses of clinical-trial results [38]. In general, only in the treatment of malignancies with a steep dose-response curve is dose intensification likely to produce significant clinical benefits. Dose intensification may be achieved by increasing the dose of one or more drugs in a combination or by decreasing the interval between treatment cycles.

Coldman and Goldie [39] have predicted that increasing dose intensity has a greater impact on eliminating sensitive cells than it does in preventing the occurrence of resistant cells. However, their model assumes that resistant cells are unaffected by treatment. If drug resistance is relative and not absolute it may be possible to increase killing of resistant cells by increasing dose. This hypothesis can be tested in the setting of minimal residual disease where clinically undetectable resistant cells remain following an initial CR to chemotherapy. Evidence showing that it is possible to overcome apparent drug resistance by increasing dose intensity is provided by studies of high-dose myeloablative therapy with bone marrow transplantation to effect hematological reconstitution. In this situation dramatic responses and long-term remissions have been reported in patients where such an outcome would be unexpected with conventional therapy. For example, for patients with very advanced lymphoma, increases in dose, particularly of alkylating agents, in the range 3- to 10-fold normal have produced significant fractions of patients who are free of disease, and in fact may be cured [40]. A similar success of salvage high-dose chemotherapy has been recently reported with a carboplatin/etoposide w/o ifosfamide combination for germ cell tumors, including patients with apparent progression of disease on primary therapy [41]. However, another important feature of the data from ABMT studies is that durable complete remissions are possible with only one or two high doses, suggesting that many of these patients were probably under-dosed during their initial treatment.

BMT is increasingly being used as salvage therapy or consolidation therapy in poor-risk patients, and the high morbidity and mortality of this approach have been reduced by advances in supportive care [42, 43]. One important advance is the use of hematopoietic growth factors. One of the main arguments for not using these types of aggressive therapies has traditionally been the very high hematological and nonhematological toxicity associated with them, which often resulted in 10–20% of iatrogenic deaths.

The introduction of hemopoietic growth factors to speed up recovery following ABMT, and the judicious use of growth-factor-primed circulating progenitor cells have led to a marked decrease in hematological toxicity and infectious complications [44, 45]. Following an initial report by Socinski et al. [46], who described 18-fold increases in the numbers of circulating myeloid progenitors (GM-CFUs) after chemotherapy alone and up to 60-fold rises when GM-CSF was added, Gianni et al. [47] described the harvesting by leukopharesis of circulating progenitor cells following high-dose cyclophosphamide and GM-CSF, and their use to speed up bone marrow recovery. The most useful contribution of circulating progenitors is probably the sparing effect on platelet transfusions: in a study reported by Sheridan et al. [48], autologous circulating progenitor cells collected during the continuous subcutaneous infusion of G-CSF alone (without chemotherapy) drastically reduced platelet recovery time in patients treated with high-dose chemotherapy (cyclophosphamide and busulphan) and ABMT. While we wait for a putative recombinant human hemopoietic growth factor selective for megakaryocyte proliferation and differentiation, circulating progenitor cells are a valid therapeutic technique, although their specific indications need to be better defined. The absence of suitable platelet donors, the development of antiplatelet antibodies or the presence of bone marrow infiltration by tumor cells might be some potential indications, although it seems that circulating tumor cells are not uncommon contaminants of leukaphoresis products [49].

## Rationale for the Use of G-CSF to Increase the Dose Intensity of Treatment

The in vivo proliferating activity of normal bone marrow cells is much higher than that of most human tumors, hence the bone marrow toxicity of cytotoxic antitumor agents has been the main dose-limiting variable. Many of the successes of combination chemotherapy can be attributed to the achievement of a higher equivalent cytotoxic dose by the combination of drugs with primarily nonoverlapping toxic effects. This led Simon and Korn [50] to develop a methodology to select optimal drug combinations based on a knowledge of their relative potencies and maximally tolerated doses. There is also increasing consensus that it is preferable to use two or three good drugs at full dose and maximum individual dose intensities, than more drugs at lower dose intensity because of toxicities.

If dose intensity is to be increased by decreasing the interval between chemotherapy cycles it would appear to be more logical to use G-CSF than GM-CSF because of its more rapid effect [6]. Clinical studies have already demonstrated the feasibility of using G-CSF or GM-CSF to allow delivery of high-dose chemotherapy without BMT, and initial results appear promising. G-CSF was used to increase the intensity of doxorubicin in patients with breast and ovarian cancer by both increasing the dose and reducing the interval between cycles [29]. With this approach it was possible to escalate the doxorubicin dose intensity 4.5-fold before reaching nonhematological dose-limiting effects. A high response rate was reported, but the duration of remission was disappointingly short. However, this 'accelerated' approach could help to shorten several combination chemotherapies or sequential therapies (like adriamycin-CMF) provided due attention is paid to cumulative thrombocytopenia and mucositis.

An EORTC study has established that G-CSF enables a shorter interval between epirubicin (100 mg/m$^2$)/cyclophosphamide (830 mg/m$^2$) treatment cycles, resulting in an increased dose intensity in patients with metastatic breast cancer [51]. The interval between chemotherapy cycles was reduced from 22 to 13 days, with G-CSF given on days 2–11 in the maximally tolerated schedule. The clinical response rate was 94% (CR 25%).

Preliminary trials with dose-intensive chemotherapy have provided encouraging results, but although high response rates have been reported, it is still too early to draw any firm conclusions. Furthermore, these trials have already revealed some limitations in using hematopoietic growth factors to increase dose intensity, for example, an increase in nonhematological toxicity and an increased risk of thrombocytopenia associated with higher doses of chemotherapy. Larger, well-designed and carefully conducted prospective studies are now needed to establish whether the wider application of high-dose therapies can lead to clinically significant results. The design of these studies is not going to be easy, considering the number of variables potentially involved: dose, intervals, single-agent chemotherapy vs. combination regimens, patient population, total dose of cytotoxics, pharmacokinetics at the high doses, adjuvant situations or advanced disease. In some preclinical animal tumor models (e.g., the rat mammary adenocarcinoma 16/C treated with adriamycin) the correlation between relative dose intensity and CR rate is better than the correlation between cumulative total dose and CR rate; but in the same tumor model the correlation between the overall duration of response and relative dose intensity is worse than the correlation between total cumulative dose and duration of response. Skipper [37] concludes a recent review on the relative merits of dose intensity versus total dose of chemotherapy by saying that, at least in animal models, dose intensity is the dominant treatment design variable with respect to the degree of therapeutic response (cure or nearness to cure); on the other hand, total dose often, but not always, correlates best with the duration of response or time to progression in animals not cured by chemotherapy.

An additional problem, of a rather different kind, is which control population should be used in randomized phase III studies. If, for example, the high-dose pilot studies suggest a 3-year survival of 70-80% (as seems to be the case for several high-dose protocols in stage II/III breast cancer patients with more than 10 positive axillary nodes), whereas historical controls fall to about 30% figures, is it realistic to expect high accrual of patients in a comparative prospective study? And yet these randomized phase III studies seem necessary to confirm that the high-dose approach can be safely regarded as 'standard' therapy. In the absence of better cytotoxic drugs or of mechanisms to ocercome drug resistance, the dose-intensity approach ought to be extensively explored to achieve the main goal of clinical oncologists: to increase the survival of cancer patients. At least two major obstacles are to be expected: the nonhematological toxicities of cytotoxic drugs, which may become dose-limiting after an increase in dose by only 2- or 3-fold for some drugs; and the biology of the tumor itself, including its propensity to molecular drug resistance, its cellular kinetics and its ability to elicit some form of immune control by the host on any remaining subclinical population of tumor cells.

### ABMT and Circulating Progenitor Cells

G-CSF and GM-CSF may be used to reduce the morbidity of very high-dose therapy with ABMT and thus may widen the applicability of this procedure. Several clinical trials have shown that hematopoietic growth factor therapy significantly accelerates ANC recovery and this is associated with a reduction in infectious complications [52]. It is important to emphasize that the use of hematopoietic growth factors in BMT does not eliminate the initial period of absolute neutropenia (the first week or 10 days following conventional ABMT) and will not allow further dose increase because the dose-limiting toxicity is nonhematological. Despite these limitations, hematopoietic growth factors represent a significant advance in the BMT setting. It remains to be determined whether the reduction in morbidity associated with G-CSF or GM-CSF translates into improved overall survival, but several groups have already experienced a marked reduction in the incidence and severity of late systemic fungal infections.

As already mentioned, hematopoietic progenitor cells mobilized from the bone marrow can be collected from peripheral blood by leukapheresis and used as an alternative or adjunct to ABMT following myeloablative therapy. Mobilization of peripheral blood progenitor cells (PBPC) by G-CSF or GM-CSF is significantly more effective than the previous approach using cyclophosphamide. Collection of PBPC following treatment with a hematopoietic growth factor is an easier, less expensive and better tolerated procedure than collecting bone marrow. An additional benefit is that theoretically there is less risk of tumor contamination in PBPC than in bone marrow. Sheridan et al. [53] treated patients with high-dose chemotherapy followed by BMT and daily administration of G-CSF. One series of patients also received G-CSF-stimulated PBPC collected prior to chemotherapy. The addition of PBPC was associated with a significant acceleration in platelet recovery compared with BMT plus G-CSF. Neutrophil recovery was similar in patients with and without PBPC, but in both groups recovery was faster than in historical controls who received BMT only.

A novel high-dose sequential regimen involving the use of CSFs and PBPC has been developed in patients with breast cancer and more than ten axillary lymph nodes at presentation, by Gianni et al. [54]. PBPC harvested after treatment with GM-CSF and cyclophosphamide were reinfused together with bone marrow following high-dose chemotherapy with L-PAM. Between the high-dose cyclophosphamide and L-PAM, the patients received vincristine, high-dose methotrexate and cisplatin sequentially, and the overall duration of treatment was about 2 months. Hematological toxicity was manageable and rapid platelet recovery was reported. At an actuarial follow-up of 2 years, results compare favorably with historical controls or sequential adriamycin-CMF, but, as already mentioned, before this type of high-dose sequential treatment is accepted as standard therapy for this high-risk group of patients, prospective studies and a longer follow-up are needed. Similarly, Peters et al. [55] have recently reported preliminary results for a high-dose study (with cyclophosphamide, cisplatin and carmustine following induction with four courses of high-dose CAF) also in breast cancer patients with more than ten axillary lymph nodes. Again, patients were rescued with G-CSF-primed PBPC and bone marrow, and iatrogenic deaths (about 12% prior to the introduction of G-CSF) decreased to a more acceptable figure of 2%. Disease-free survival at 2 years was about 72% (as compared to 24–31% of historical controls), and a randomized phase III study is now in progress to verify these encouraging results.

Clearly, the use of PBPC is a promising approach for delivering high-dose chemotherapy more safely. However, the technique remains experimental and further studies are required. There are probably enough pilot studies (and consensus) to concentrate on comparative phase III studies looking for survival advantage in high-risk populations of patients with chemosensitive malignancies. In my view, more pilot studies of this kind can only be justified if truly innovative, or if carried out by experimental hematologists with the aims of improving the technique, lowering costs, or both (for example, the 'in vitro' expansion of progenitor cells prior to reinfusion, or the identification and isolation of true pluripotent human stem cells with self-renewing potential). If the initial encouraging results are verified, the use of PBPC may eventually supersede BMT and thus make high-dose chemotherapy a possibility for a larger number of patients.

## References


1 Bodey GP, Buckley M, Sathe YS, Freireich EJ: Quantitative relationships between circulating leukocytes and infection in patients with acute leukemia. Ann Intern Med 1966;64:328–340.
2 De Vita VT: Principles of chemotherapy; in DeVita VT, Hellman S, Rosenberg SA (eds): Cancer Principles and Practice of Oncology. Philadelphia, Lippincott, 1989, pp 276–300.
3 Bronchud MH: Hemopoietic growth factors: Unravelling the secrets of blood formation. Eur J Cancer 1991;27:372–376.
4 Morstyn G, Sheridan WP: Colony-stimulating factors in cancer therapy; in Pinedo HM, Longo DL, Chabner BA (eds): Cancer Chemotherapy and Biological Response Modifiers, Annual 13. Amsterdam, Elsevier 1992, pp 308–326.
5 Platzer E: Human hematopoietic growth factors. Eur J Haematol 1989;42:1–15.
6 Lord BI, Bronchud MH, Owens S, et al: The kinetics of human granulopoiesis following treatment with granulocyte colony-stimulating factor in vivo. Proc Natl Acad Sci USA 1989; 86:9499–9503.
7 Lord BI, Gurney H, Chang J, et al: Haemopoietic cell kinetics in humans treated with rGM-CSF. Int J Cancer 1992;50:26–31.
8 Groopman JE, Molina M, Scadden DT: Hematopoietic growth factors. New Engl J Med 1989; 321:1449–1459.
9 Gabrilove J: The development of granulocyte colony-stimulating factor in its various clinical applications. Blood 1992;80:1382–1385.
10 Bronchud MH, Scarffe JH, Thatcher N, et al: Phase I/II study of recombinant human granulocyte colony-stimulating factor in patients receiving intensive chemotherapy for small cell lung cancer. Br J Cancer 1987;56:809–813.
11 Morstyn G, Campbell L, Souza LM, et al: Effect of granulocyte colony-stimulating factor on neutropenia induced by cytotoxic chemotherapy. Lancet 1988;i:667–672.
12 Gabrilove JL, Jakubowski A, Scher J, et al: Effect of granulocyte colony-stimulating factor on neutropenia and associated morbidity due to the chemotherapy for transitional cell carcinoma of the urothelium. New Engl J Med 1988; 318:1414–1422.
13 Neidhart J, Mangalik A, Kohler W, et al: Granulocyte colony-stimulating factor stimulates recovery of granulocytes in patients receiving dose intensive chemotherapy without bone marrow transplantation. J Clin Oncol 1989;7: 1685–1692.
14 Bronchud MH, Howell A, Crowther D, et al: The use of granulocyte colony-stimulating factor to increase the intensity of treatment with doxorubicin in patients with advanced breast and ovarian cancer. Br J Cancer 1989;60:121–125.
15 Crawford J, Ozer H, Stoller R, et al: Reduction by granulocyte colony-stimulating factor of fever and neutropenia induced by chemotherapy in patients with small cell lung cancer. New Engl J Med 1991;325:164–170.
16 Green JA, Trillet VN, Manegold C, et al: G-CSF with CDE chemotherapy in small cell lung cancer: Interim results from a randomized, placebo-controlled trial (Abstract 832). Proc Am Soc Clin Oncol 1991;10:243.
17 Sagarra A, Bronchud MH: Toxicity of hematopoietic growth factors. Forum 1992;24:4–18.
18 Hornung RL, Longo DL: Hematopoietic stem cell depletion by restorative growth factor regimens during repeated high-dose cyclophosphamide therapy. Blood 1992;80:77–83.
19 Moore MAS: Does stem cell exhaustion result from combining hematopoietic growth factors with chemotherapy? If so, how do we prevent it? Blood 1992;80:3–7.
20 Lindemann A, Herrmann F, Oster W, et al: Hematologic effects of recombinant human granulocyte colony-stimulating factor in patients with malignancy. Blood 1989;74:2644–2651.
21 Bronchud MH, Potter MR, Morgenstern G, et al: In vitro and in vivo analysis of the effects of recombinant human granulocyte colony-stimulating factor in patients. Br J Cancer 1988;58: 64–69.
22 Bronchud MH, Dexter TM: Clinical use of hematopoietic growth factors. Blood Rev 1989; 3:66–70.
23 Peters WP, Stuart A, Affronti ML, et al: Neutrophil migration is defective during recombinant human granulocyte colony-stimulating factor infusion after autologous bone marrow transplantation in humans. Blood 1988;72: 1310–1315.
24 Dedhar S, Galloway P, Eaves C: Human granulocyte-macrophage colony-stimulating factor is a growth factor for a variety of cell types of non hemopoietic origin. Proc Am Soc Clin Oncol 1988;29:51.
25 Ohno R, Tomonaga M, Kobayashi T, et al: Effect of granulocyte colony-stimulating factor after intensive induction therapy in relapsed or refractory acute leukemia. New Engl J Med 1990;323:871–877.
26 Lieschke GJ, Ramenghi U, O'Connor MP, et al: Studies of oral neutrophil levels in patients receiving G-CSF after autologous marrow transplantation. Br J Haematol 1992;82:589–595.
27 Blayney DW, Williams S, Mortimer J, et al: Neupogen (r-metHuG-CSF) ameliorates neutropenia during CHOP chemotherapy. ASCO Proc 1992, 320 (abstract 1088).
28 Pettengell R, Gurney H, Radford J, et al: A randomised trial of recombinant human granulocyte colony-stimulating factor to preserve dose-intensity in non-Hodgkin's lymphoma (abstract 1083). Proc Am Soc Clin Ontol 1992;11: 319.
29 Bronchud MH, Howell A, Crowther D, et al: The use of granulocyte colony-stimulating factor to increase the intensity of treatment with doxorubicin in patients with advanced breast and ovarian cancer. Br J Cancer 1989;60:121–125.
30 Steinke B, Manegold C, Freund M, et al: G-CSF for treatment intensification in high-grade malignant non-Hodgkin's lymphomas. Onkologie 1992;15:46–50.
31 Cabanillas F: To CHOP or not to CHOP ... is that the question? (editorial) Ann Oncol 1992; 3:183–185.
32 Fisher RI, Gaynor E, Dahlberg S, et al: A phase III comparison of CHOP vs. m-BACOD vs. ProMACE-CytaBOM vs. MACOP-B in patients with intermediate or high-grade non-Hodgkin's lymphoma: Preliminary results of SWOG-8516, The National High-Priority Lymphoma Study (abstract 1067). Proc Am Soc Clin Oncol 1992;11:315.
33 Furman WL, Fairclough DL, Huhn RD, et al: Therapeutic effects and pharmacokinetics of recombinant human granulocyte-macrophage colony-stimulating factor in childhood cancer patients receiving myelosuppressive chemotherapy. J Clin Oncol 1991;9:1022–1028.
34 Stute N, Santana VM, Rodman JH, et al: Pharmacokinetics of subcutaneous recombinant human granulocyte colony-stimulating factor in children. Blood 1992;79:2849–2854.
35 Fukuda M, Kojima S, Matsumoto K, et al: Autotransplantation of peripheral blood stem cells mobilized by chemotherapy and recombinant human granulocyte colony-stimulating factor in childhood neuroblastoma and non-Hodgkin's lymphoma. Br J Haematol 1992;80: 327–331.
36 Fushiki M, Abe M: Randomized double-blinded controlled study of rhG-CF in patients with neutropenia induced by radiation therapy (abstract 1437). Proc Am Soc Clin Oncol 1992; 11:410.
37 Skipper H: Dose intensity versus total dose of chemotherapy: An experimental basis; in DeVita VT, Hellman S, Rosenberg SA (eds): Important Advances in Oncology. Philadelphia, Lippincott, 1990, pp 43–64.
38 Hryniuk W, Bush H: The importance of dose intensity in chemotherapy of metastatic breast cancer. J Clin Oncol 1984;2:1281–1290.
39 Coldman AJ, Goldie JH: Impact of dose-intense chemotherapy on the development of permanent drug resistance. Semin Oncol 1987; 14:29–33.
40 Antman K, Eder JP, Frei E III: High-dose chemotherapy with bone marrow support for solid tumors, in DeVita VT, Hellman S, Rosenberg SA (eds): Important Advances in Oncology. Philadelphia, Lippincott, 1987, pp 221–232.
41 Rosti G, Albertazzi L, Salvioni R, et al: High-dose chemotherapy supported with autologous bone marrow transplantation (ABMT) in germ cell tumors: A phase two study. Ann Oncol 1992;3:809–812.
42 Carella AM, Carlier P, Congiu A, et al: Autologous bone marrow transplantation as adjuvant treatment for high risk Hodgkin's disease in first complete remission after MOPP/ABVD protocol. Bone Marrow Transplant 1991;8:99–103.

43 Goldstone AH, McMillan AK: Conceptual problems in relation to dose escalation in the first remission Hodgkin's disease. Ann Oncol 1992;3(suppl 4):91–93.
44 Nemunaitis J, Singer JW, Buckner CD, et al: Use of recombinant human granulocyte-macrophage colony-stimulating factor in autologous marrow transplantation of lymphoid malignancies. Blood 1988;72:834–836.
45 Sheridan WP, Morstyn G, Wolf M, et al: Granulocyte colony-stimulating factor and neutrophil recovery after high-dose chemotherapy and autologous bone marrow transplantation. Lancet 1989;ii:891–895.
46 Socinski MA, Cannistra SA, Elias A, et al: Granulocyte-macrophage colony-stimulating factor expands the circulating haemopoietic progenitor cell compartment in man. Lancet 1988;i:1194–1198.
47 Gianni AM, Siena S, Bregni M, et al: Granulocyte-macrophage colony-stimulating factor to harvest circulating hematopoietic stem cells for autotransplantation. Lancet 1989;ii:580–584.
48 Sheridan WP, Begley CG, Juttner CA, et al: Effect of peripheral-blood progenitor cells mobilised by filgrastim (G-CSF) on platelet recovery after high-dose chemotherapy. Lancet 1992;i:640–644.
49 Hardingham JE, Kotasek D, Dobrovic A, et al: Detection of minimal residual tumor cells in non-Hodgkin's lymphoma (NHL) stem cell harvests using molecular markers (abstract 1190). Proc Am Assoc Cancer Res 1992;11:199.
50 Simon R, Korn EL: Selecting drug combinations based on total equivalent dose (dose intensity). J Natl Cancer Inst 1990;82:1469–1476.
51 Piccart M, van der Schueren E, Bruning P, et al: High-dose intensity chemotherapy with epiadriamycin, cyclophosphamide and rh-met-HuG-CSF in breast cancer patients (abstract 308). Eur J Cancer 1991;27(suppl 2).
52 Mertelsmann R, Peters W: Hematopoietic Growth Factors. Educational Book. Am Soc Clin Oncol Meet Houston, 1991.
53 Sheridan WP, Begley CG, Juttner CA, et al: Effect of peripheral blood progenitor cells mobilised by filgrastim (G-CSF) on platelet recovery after high-dose chemotherapy. Lancet 1992;339:640–644.
54 Gianni AM, Siena S, Bregni M, et al: Growth-factor supported high-dose sequential adjuvant chemotherapy in breast cancer with >10 positive nodes (abstract 68). Proc Am Soc Clin Oncol 1992;11:60.
55 Peters WP, Ross M, Vredenburgh J, et al: High-dose alkylating agents and autologous bone marrow support for stage II/III breast cancer involving ten or more axillary lymph nodes (abstract 59). Proc Am Soc Clin Oncol 1992;11:58.

Oncology 1994;51:198–204

*Kazuo Motoyoshi*

The Third Department of Internal Medicine, National Defense Medical College, Saitama, Japan

# Macrophage Colony-Stimulating Factor for Cancer Therapy

**Key Words**

Macrophage colony-stimulating factor
Cancer chemotherapy
Quality of life
Tumor necrosis factor
Reactive nitrogen intermediates

**Abstract**

Macrophage colony-stimulating factor (M-CSF) is a homodimeric glycoprotein which stimulates differentiation of progenitor cells to mature monocytes and enhances production of hemopoietic growth factors from mature monocytes such as granulocyte-macrophage CSF, granulocyte CSF and megakaryocyte potentiator, suggesting that M-CSF administration enhances production of monocytes, neutrophils and platelets. Since the commercial availability of M-CSF in 1991, serial M-CSF infusions at a daily dose of 8 million units have been performed in patients with acute myeloid leukemia in complete remission after combination chemotherapy. Although M-CSF infusion reduced the duration of neutropenia in 3 of 5 patients, it reduced the duration of pyrexia over 37 °C in all patients, and that over 38 °C in 4 of 5 patients. Average durations of pyrexia and parenteral antibiotic injections were significantly shorter in M-CSF than in control courses. Although M-CSF infusion reduced the duration of thrombopenia in 2 of 5 patients, it reduced total platelet units transfused in 4 of 5 patients. The average number of platelet units transfused after combination chemotherapy was significantly lower in M-CSF than in control courses. In mice, M-CSF injection increased the serum concentration of reactive nitrogen intermediates which inhibited the growth of L1210 cells, and increased the survival rate of mice previously injected with them. These results indicate that M-CSF may be a promising agent not for improving patients' quality of life after cancer chemotherapy, but also in cancer immunotherapy.

## Introduction

Macrophage colony-stimulating factor (M-CSF) has been shown to stimulate monocyte progenitor cells to differentiate to mature monocytes [1], and the latter to produce several hematopoietic growth factors such as granulocyte-macrophage CSF (GM-CSF) [2], granulocyte CSF (G-CSF) [2] and megakaryocyte potentiator (Meg-POT [3]. Human M-CSF thus augmented the production of monocytes, neutrophils and platelets in bone marrow when it was injected to cancer-bearing patients after cancer chemotherapy [3, 4]. In addition to hematopoiesis-stimulating activity, M-CSF acts to enhance differentiation of cytotrophoblasts to syncytiotrophoblasts which produce and secrete human chorionic gonadotropin [5], and also enhances low-density-lipoprotein receptor (LDL-R)-dependent as well as -independent clearance of plasma cholesterol in patients with chronic neutropenia [6] and normal rabbits [7], and LDL-R-independent clearance in LDL-R-deficient rabbits (Watanabe heritable hyperlipi-

Kazuo Motoyoshi, MD
The Third Department of Internal Medicine
National Defense Medical College
3-2 Namiki, Tokorozawa-shi
Saitama-ken 359 (Japan)


0030–2414/94/0512–0198
$5.00/0

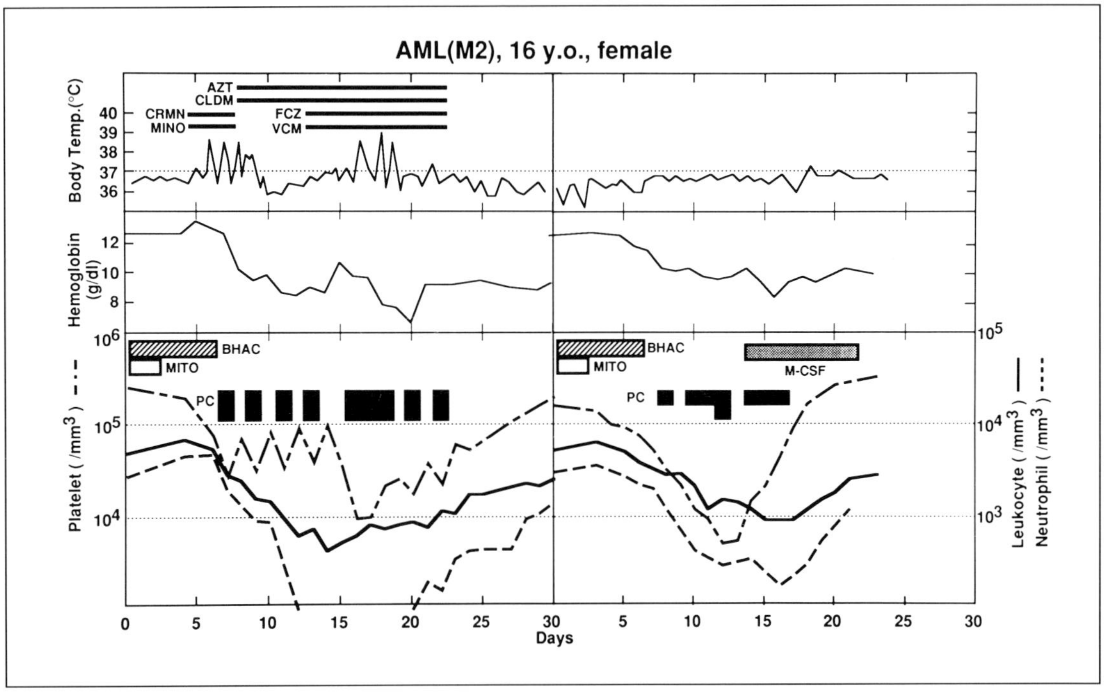


**Fig. 1.** Clinical course of a patient with AML(M2) in complete remission. Infusion with M-CSF markedly accelerated hematopoietic recovery, and reduced durations of pyrexia and parenteral antibiotic injections and also reduced total units of platelet concentrate (PC) transfused. AZT = Aztreonam; CLDM = clindamycin hydrochloride; CRMN = carumonam sodium; FCZ = fluconazole; MINO = minocycline hydrochloride; VCM = vancomycin hydrochloride; BHAC = behenoylcytosine arabinoside; MITO = mitoxantrone.

demic strain) [7]. M-CSF definitely prevented the progression of atherosclerosis in Watanabe rabbits [8]. In a strain of osteopetrotic mutant mice, op/op, a point mutation was found in the structural gene of M-CSF which resulted in the production of an inactive amino-terminal fragment of M-CSF molecule [9]. Our previous in vitro experiments demonstrated that M-CSF enhanced an antibody-dependent tumor-killing activity of human monocytes against a lymphocytic leukemia cell line. Raji, through an increment in Fc receptor site number on the monocyte surface which resulted in a higher frequency of monocyte attachment to antibody-bound tumor cells [10]. M-CSF also enhanced antibody-independent tumor-killing activity of monocytes against several human leukemic cell lines such as HL60, U937, K562 and Daudi in vitro, in which tumor necrosis factor (TNF) was suggested to be somewhat involved because the addition of anti-TNF-antibody partially neutralized the tumor-killing activity of monocytes [11]. It has recently been reported that monocytes have two killing mechanisms against tumor cells [12, 13]: one is TNF and the other reactive nitrogen intermediates (RNI). Our preliminary experiments demonstrated that mice given M-CSF 3 h before triggering by lipopolysaccharide (LPS) injection had a higher concentration of TNF in their serum, and injection of M-CSF enhanced RNI production by macrophages and increased the serum concentration of RNI. In addition to these biological activities, we recently found that M-CSF infusion markedly improved patients' quality of life, reducing periods with pyrexia or the requirement for blood transfusion after cancer chemotherapy.

## Clinical Courses of Leukemic Patients Treated with M-CSF

Since M-CSF became commercially available in 1991, patients with acute nonlymphocytic leukemia or ovarian cancer after cancer chemotherapy, and patients after bone marrow transplantation have been treated with M-CSF. In our hospital, several patients with acute myeloid leukemia (AML) were treated with serial M-CSF infusion after combination chemotherapy. Figure 1 demonstrates the clinical course of a 16 year-old female patient with AML

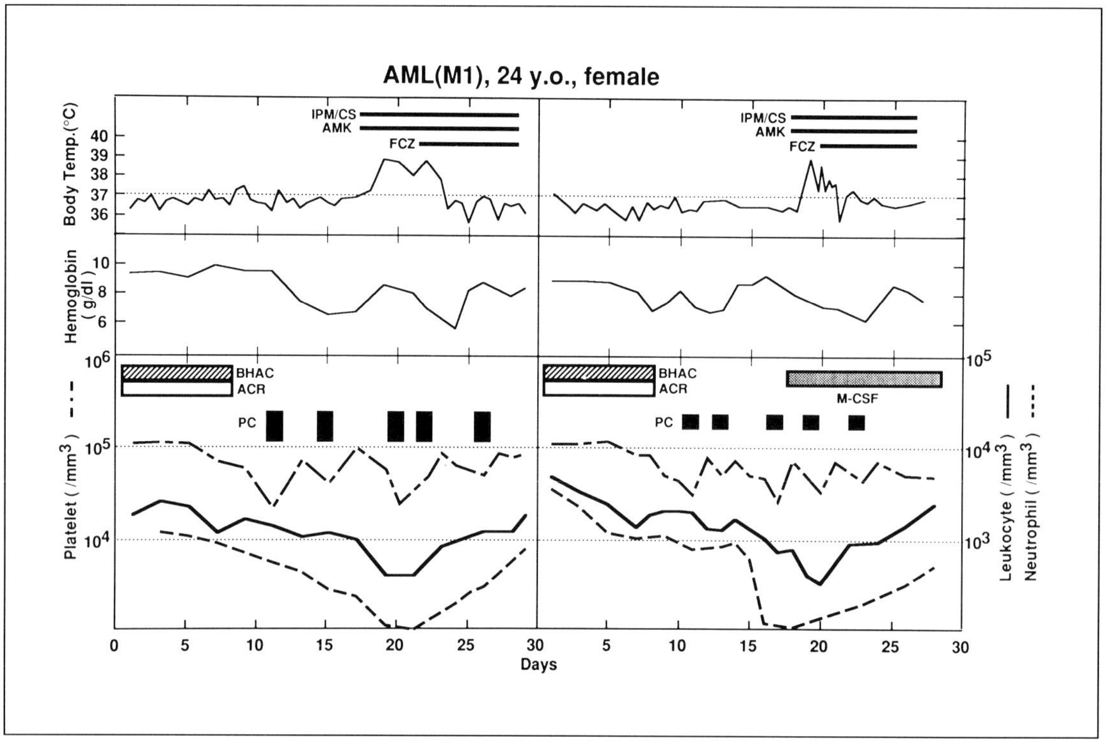


**Fig. 2.** Clinical course of a patient with AML(M1) in complete remission. Although infusion with M-CSF did not accelerate hematopoietic recovery, it reduced durations of pyrexia and parenteral-antibiotic injections and also reduced total units of PC transfused. IPM/CS = Imipenem/cilastatin sodium; AMK = amikacin sulfate; FCZ = fluconazole; BHAC = behenoylcytosine arabinoside; ACR = aclarubicin.

**Table 1.** Patient profiles

| Case | Age | Sex | Diagnosis | Combination chemotherapy |
|---|---|---|---|---|
| K.S. | 27 | M | AML(M1) in CR | BHAC<br>DNR<br>6MP |
| S.K. | 16 | F | AML(M2) in CR | BHAC<br>MITO |
| S.Y. | 60 | M | AML(M1) in CR | BHAC<br>VP16<br>VDS |
| T.O. | 27 | M | AML(M2) in CR | BHAC<br>MITO |
| Y.W. | 24 | F | AML(M1) in CR | BHAC<br>ACR |

CR = Complete remission: BHAC = behenoylcytosine arabinoside; DNR = daunorubicin; 6MP = 6-mercaptopurine; MITO = mitoxantrone; VP16 = etoposide; VDS = vindesine; ACR = aclarubicin.

(FAB:M2) in complete remission. She was treated twice with the same chemotherapeutic regimen consisting of behenoylcytosine arabinoside (BHAC) and mitoxantrone (MITO) with an interval of 21 months. She did not receive M-CSF infusion after the first chemotherapy (first course), but received it at a daily dose of 8 million units for 9 days from the 13th day after the initiation of the second chemotherapy (second course). She developed severe neutropenia during the first course, and had a fever over 38 °C because of pneumonia for 5 days during the neutrophil nadir and needed to receive several kinds of parenteral antibiotics for 17 days. She also developed severe thrombocytopenia and received 180 units of platelet concentrate (PC). On the other hand, she developed neither severe neutropenia, nor severe thrombocytopenia during the second course when she was treated with M-CSF infusion. She did not have a fever over 38 °C and received only 80 platelet units.

Figure 2 demonstrates the clinical course of a 24-year-old female patient with AML (FAB:M1) in complete

**Table 2.** Effects of M-CSF injections on durations (days) of neutropenia, pyrexia and parenteral antibiotics injections

| Case | M-CSF injections | Duration of neutropenia | | Duration of pyrexia | | Duration of parenteral antibiotic injections |
|---|---|---|---|---|---|---|
| | | <200 | <500 | >37 °C | >38 °C | |
| K.S. | – | 23 | 29 | 25 | 8 | 31 |
| | + | 17 | 25 | 18 | 3 | 12 |
| S.K. | – | 12 | 18 | 12 | 6 | 18 |
| | + | 3 | 10 | 2 | 0 | 0 |
| S.Y. | – | 9 | 12 | 4 | 1 | 7 |
| | + | 7 | 10 | 2 | 1 | 5 |
| T.O. | – | 10 | 13 | 16 | 4 | 16 |
| | + | 10 | 12 | 7 | 3 | 7 |
| Y.W. | – | 8 | 18 | 10 | 5 | 10 |
| | + | 8 | 18 | 5 | 2 | 7 |

remission. She was serially treated twice with the same chemotherapeutic regimen consisting of BHAC and aclarubicin hydrochloride (ACR). She did not receive M-CSF infusion after the first chemotherapy (first course), but received it at a daily dose of 8 million units for 11 days from the 17th day after the initiation of the second chemotherapy (second course). Although M-CSF infusion did not accelerate neutrophil recovery in this case, it reduced the duration of pyrexia over 38 °C from 5 to 2 days, suggesting that M-CSF protected the patient from infections during neutropenia. M-CSF infusion did not accelerate platelet recovery, but reduced the total platelet units transfused from 100 to 50 units. On the basis of these clinical observations, we tried to evaluate the effects of M-CSF infusion not only on hematopoietic recovery, but also on improvement in patients' quality of life such as a reduction in the duration of pyrexia, reduction in the period with antibiotic injection, and reduction in blood transfusion units after combination chemotherapies.

## Effect of M-CSF Infusion on Pyrexia during Neutropenia

Table 1 shows the clinical profiles of 5 patients with AML in complete remission who were treated with two courses of combination chemotherapy, each consisting of the same chemotherapeutic regimen, and who received M-CSF infusion in one but not in the other course. Table 2 demonstrates the duration of neutropenia below 200 or 500/mm$^3$, the duration of pyrexia over 37 or 38 °C, and the duration of parenteral antibiotic injections in control and in M-CSF-infused courses for these 5 patients. M-CSF infusion reduced the duration of neutropenia in 3 patients, and the duration of pyrexia and parenteral antibiotic injections in all 5.

Table 3 shows that M-CSF infusion significantly reduced the average duration of pyrexia over 38 or 37 °C during neutropenia below 500 or 200/mm$^3$. Interestingly, M-CSF infusion significantly reduced the average ratios of days with pyrexia over 38 or 37 °C to days with neutropenia below 500 or 200/mm$^3$. M-CSF infusion also reduced the average duration of parenteral antibiotic injections from 16.4 ± 9.3 to 6.2 ± 4.3 days ($p < 0.05$). These results clearly indicate that M-CSF infusion not only accelerated neutrophil recovery, but also protected the patients from infections during neutropenia after combination chemotherapy. Although the protective mechanism of M-CSF to infections during neutropenia is not well understood, it is possible that M-CSF enhances the killing activity of monocytes against several bacteria and fungi. We previously reported the effects of M-CSF on the reduction of viable bacteria and on survival of mice during *Listeria monocytogenes* infection [14]. Khwaja et al. [15] reported that M-CSF infusion increased the ability of monocytes to ingest and degrade *Candida*, and increased the number of monocytes entering a skin window. In a phase I clinical trial, Nemunaitis et al. [16] found that 39% of the patients with documented fungal infection and 50% of patients with presumed fungal infection survived 100 days after initiation of treatment with M-CSF, while historically comparable patients with invasive fungal disease who had not received M-CSF had a survival of less than 20%, indicating antifungal effects of M-CSF during neutropenia [16].

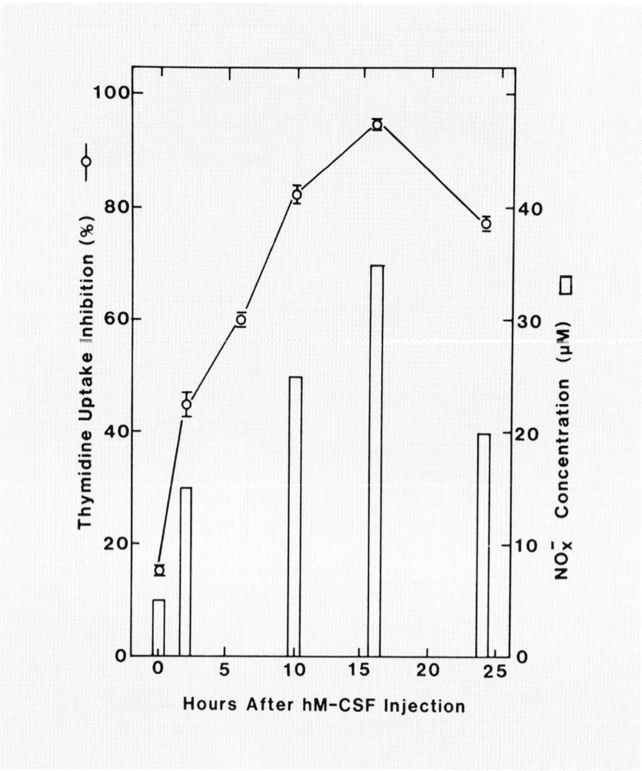


**Fig. 3.** Growth-inhibiting activity and serum $NO_x^-$ concentration of mice injected with M-CSF (100 μg/kg). Growth-inhibiting activity was measured by inhibition of thymidine uptake to L1210 cells, and concentration of $NO_x^-$ according to the method reported by Stuehr et al. [18].

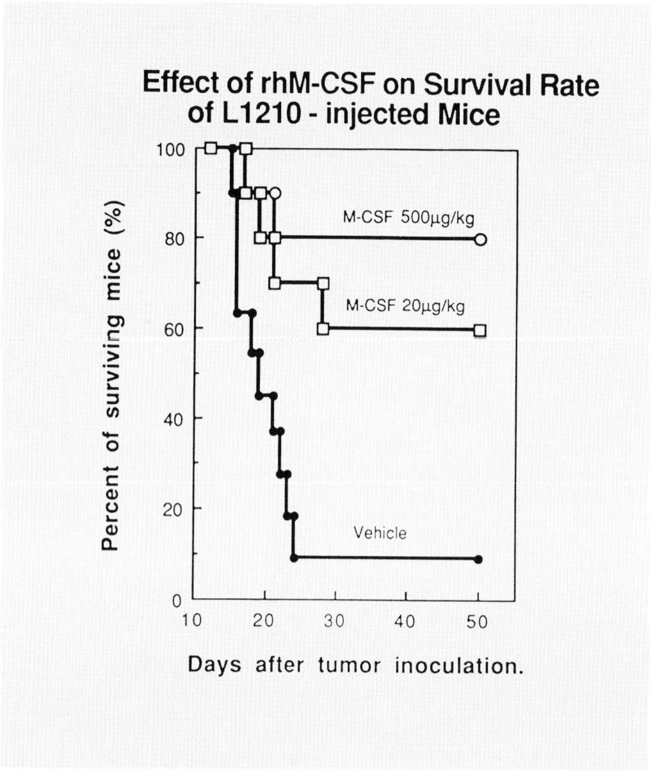


**Fig. 4.** Effect of M-CSF on survival rate of mice previously injected with a small number of L1210 cells (100 cells/mouse). M-CSF (0, 20 or 500 μg/kg) was injected for 5 days from a day after L1210 injection.

**Table 3.** Effect of M-CSF infusion on pyrexia during neutropenia

| | Control course | M-CSF-injected course | |
|---|---|---|---|
| Duration of pyrexia >38 °C during neutropenia <500/mm³, day | 3.8 ± 1.3 | 1.6 ± 1.3 | $p < 0.01$ |
| Duration of pyrexia >37 °C during neutropenia <500/mm³, day | 8.6 ± 7.1 | 4.6 ± 5.3 | $p < 0.01$ |
| Ratio of days with pyrexia >38 °C to days with neutropenia <500/mm³, % | 22.2 ± 7.1 | 10.7 ± 8.3 | $p < 0.01$ |
| Ratio of days with pyrexia >37 °C to days with neutropenia <500/mm³, % | 46.0 ± 16.9 | 27.1 ± 18.1 | $p < 0.01$ |
| Duration of pyrexia >38 °C during neutropenia <200/mm³, days | 3.8 ± 1.3 | 1.8 ± 1.3 | $p < 0.01$ |
| Duration of pyrexia >37 °C during neutropenia <200/mm³, days | 8.0 ± 6.3 | 3.6 ± 3.7 | $p < 0.05$ |
| Ratio of days with pyrexia >38 °C to days with neutropenia <200/mm³, % | 36.7 ± 20.7 | 18.1 ± 12.2 | $p < 0.05$ |
| Ratio of days with pyrexia >38 °C to days with neutropenia <200/mm³, % | 64.0 ± 22.5 | 32.1 ± 21.7 | $p < 0.01$ |

**Table 4.** Effects of M-CSF injections on the duration of thrombopenia and the total units of transfused platelets

| Case | M-CSF injections | Duration of thrombopenia ($<1 \times 10^5/mm^3$) days | Total units of platelets transfused |
|---|---|---|---|
| S.K. | – | 21 | 180 |
| | + | 12 | 90 |
| T.O. | – | 22 | 100 |
| | + | 17 | 40 |
| K.S. | – | 29 | 120 |
| | + | 28 | 90 |
| Y.W. | – | 29 | 100 |
| | + | 29 | 50 |
| S.Y. | – | 20 | 20 |
| | + | 22 | 30 |

## Effect of M-CSF Infusion on Platelet Transfusion during Thrombopenia

Table 4 shows the duration of thrombocytopenia below $1 \times 10^5/mm^3$, and the total platelet units transfused. M-CSF injections reduced the duration of thrombopenia in only 2 patients, but reduced the total platelet units transfused in 4 patients. The average total platelet units transfused in the M-CSF-infused course was $60.0 \pm 28.3$ units, significantly lower than in the control course ($104.0 \pm 57.3$ units; $p < 0.05$). Khwaja et al. [17] conducted a clinical study in which the effect of M-CSF on hematopoietic recovery after autologous bone marrow transplantation was evaluated, and found that M-CSF patients receiving $>2 \times 10^8$ mononuclear cells/kg body weight became platelet-transfusion-independent by day 17 (control 29: $p < 0.05$) and reached a platelet count of $5 \times 10^4/mm^3$ by day 21 (control 40; $p < 0.05$). We also reported that M-CSF injections accelerated the recovery not only from neutropenia, but also from thrombocytopenia after cancer chemotherapy [4].

## Cancer Immunotherapy with M-CSF

Since M-CSF enhances the tumor-killing activity of monocytes [10, 11], it is hoped that M-CSF may be used alone or in combination with anticancer drugs for cancer treatment (cancer immunotherapy). In a preliminary experiment using mice, we found that M-CSF injection increased serum levels of RNI which suppressed the growth of murine lymphocytic leukemia cells (L1210) (fig. 3), and increased the survival rate of mice previously injected with a small number of L1210 cells (100 cells/mouse, fig. 4), indicating that M-CSF could be useful as an immunotherapeutic agent in the treatment of chemotherapy-resistant cancer, in the prevention of metastasis [19], and in the prevention of relapse after bone marrow transplant [20], or in the treatment of myelodysplastic syndrome.

## References


1 Motoyoshi K, Takaku F, Mizoguchi H, Miura Y: Purification and some properties of colony-stimulating factor from normal human urine. Blood 1978;52:1012–1020.

2 Motoyoshi K, Yoshida K, Hatake K, Saito M, Miura Y, Yanai N, Yamada M, Kawashima T, Wong GG, Temple PA, Leary AC, Witek-Giannoti JS, Fujisawa M, Yuo A, Okabe T, Takaku F: Recombinant and native human urinary colony-stimulating factor directly augments granulocytic and granulocyte-macrophage colony-stimulating factor production of human peripheral blood monocytes. Exp Hematol 1989;17:68–71.

3 Motoyoshi K, Yoshida K, Yanai N, Takaku F: Role of human monocytic colony-stimulating factor in hematopoiesis; in Kawade Y, Kobayashi S (eds): The Biology of the Interferon System, 1988. Tokyo, Kodansha Scientific, 1989, pp 253–258.

4 Motoyoshi K, Takaku F: Human monocytic colony-stimulating factor (hM-CSF), phase I/II clinical studies; in Mertelsmann R, Herrman F (eds): Hematopoietic Growth Factors in Clinical Applications. New York, Dekker, 1990, pp 161–175.

5 Saito S, Saito M, Motoyoshi K, Ichijo M: Enhancing effects of human macrophage colony-stimulating factor on the secretion of human chorionic gonadotropin by human chorionic villous cells and tPA-30-1 cells. Biochem Biophys Res Commun 1991;178:1099–1104.

6 Motoyoshi K, Takaku F: Serum cholesterol-lowering activity of human monoytic colony-stimulating factor. Lancet 1989;ii:326–327.

7 Shimano H, Yamada N, Ishibashi S, Harada K, Matsumoto A, Mori N, Inaba T, Motoyoshi K, Itakura H, Takaku F: Human monocytic colony-stimulating factor enhances the clearance of lipoproteins containing apolipoprotein B100 via both low density lipoprotein receptor-dependent and -independent pathways in rabbits. J Biol Chem 1990;265:12869–12875.

8 Inoue I, Inaba T, Motoyoshi K, Harada K, Shimano H, Kawamura M, Gotohda T, Oka T, Shiomi M, Watanabe Y, Tsukada T, Yazaki Y, Takaku F, Yamada N: Macrophage colony-stimulating factor prevents the progression of atherosclerosis in Watanabe heritable hyperlipidemic rabbits. Atherosclerosis 1992;93:245–254.

9 Yoshida H, Hayashi S, Kunisada T, Ogawa M, Nishikawa S, Okamura H, Sudo T, Shultz LD, Nishikawa S: The murine mutation osteopetrosis is in the coding region of the macrophage colony-stimulating factor gene. Nature 1990; 345:442–443.
10 Suzu S, Yanai N, Saito M, Kawashima T, Saito M, Takaku F, Motoyoshi K: Enhancement of the antibody-dependent tumoricidal activity of human monocytes by human monocytic colony-stimulating factor. Jpn J Cancer Res 1990; 81:79–84.
11 Suzu S, Yokota H, Yamada M, Yanai N, Saito M, Kawashima T, Saito M, Takaku F, Motoyoshi K: Enhancing effect of human monocytic colony-stimulating factor on monocyte tumoricidal activity. Cancer Res 1989;49:5913–5917.
12 Hasday JD, Shah EM, Lieberman P: Macrophage tumor necrosis factor release is induced by contact with some tumors. J Immunol 1990; 145:371–379.
13 Higuchi M, Higashi N, Taki H, Osawa S: Cytolytic mechanisms of activated macrophages. Tumor necrosis factor and *l*-arginine-dependent mechanisms act synergistically as the major cytolytic mechanisms of activated macrophages. J Immunol 1990;144:1425–1431.
14 Kayashima S, Tsuru S, Shinomiya N, Katsura Y, Motoyoshi K, Rokutanda M, Nagata N: Effects of macrophage colony-stimulating factor on reduction of viable bacteria and survival of mice during *Listeria monocytogenes* infection: Characteristics of monocyte subpopulations. Infect Immun 1991;59:4677–4680.
15 Khwaja A, Johnson B, Addison IE, Yong K, Ruthven K, Abramson S, Linch DC: In vivo effects of macrophage colony-stimulating factor on human monocyte function. Br J Haematol 1991;77:25–31.
16 Nemunaitis JD, Meyer CD, Buckner K, Shennon-Dorcy, M, Shulman H, Bianco JA, Higano CS, Groves E, Storb R, Hansen J, Appelbaum FR, Singer JW: Phase I trial of recombinant human macrophage colony-stimulating factor in patients with invasive fungal infections. Blood 1991;78:907–913.
17 Khwaja A, Yong K, Jones M, Chopra R, McMillan AK, Goldstone AH, Patterson KG, Matheson C, Ruthven K, Abramson SB, Linch DC: The effect of macrophage colony-stimulating factor on haematopoietic recovery after autologous bone marrow transplantation. Br J Haematol 1992;81:288–295.
18 Stuehr DJ, Marletta MA: Mammarian nitrate biosynthesis: Mouse macrophages produce nitrite and nitrate in response to *Escherichia coli* lipopolysaccharide. Proc Natl Acad Sci USA 1985;82:7738–7742.
19 Hume DA, Donahue RE, Fidler I: The therapeutic effect of human recombinant macrophage colony stimulating factor (CSF-1) in experimental murine metastatic melanoma. Lymphokine Res 1989;8:69–77.
20 Masaoka T, Shibata H, Ohno R, Katoh S, Harada M, Motoyoshi K, Takaku F, Sakuma A: Double blind test of human urinary macrophage colony-stimulating factor for allogeneic and syngeneic bone marrow transplantation: Effectiveness of treatment and 2-year follow-up for relapse of leukemia. Br J Haematol 1990; 76:501–505.

Oncology 1994;51:205–214

*George Morstyn*[a]
*Sherri Brown*[a]
*Michael Gordon*[b]
*Jeffrey Crawford*[c]
*George Demetri*[d]
*William Rich*[a]
*Brian McGuire*[a]
*MaryAnn Foote*[a]
*Ian McNiece*[a]

[a] Amgen Inc., Thousand Oaks, Calif.;
[b] Indiana University Medical Center, Indianapolis, Ind.;
[c] Duke University, Durham, N.C., and
[d] Dana-Farber Cancer Institute, Boston, Mass., USA

# Stem Cell Factor Is a Potent Synergistic Factor in Hematopoiesis

**Key Words**
Stem cell factor
r-metHuSCF
Synergistic action
Clinical studies
Preclinical studies
Peripheral blood progenitor cell mobilization
Lethal-irradiation protection

**Abstract**
Stem cell factor (SCF), a ligand for c-*kit,* has a broad range of activities including effects on cells at or near the level of the multipotential stem cell as well as on committed cells. Preclinical studies show that SCF can protect against lethal irradiation, elicit multilineage responses in peripheral blood and bone marrow cellularity, and increase circulating peripheral blood progenitor cells (PBPC) in a dose-dependent manner. Recombinant human SCF has major clinical potential through its synergy with other factors, especially recombinant human granulocyte colony-stimulating factor, to enhance mobilization of PBPC.

## Introduction

A complex, tightly regulated process controls production of the hematopoietic progenitor cells committed to different cell lineages from a common precursor cell. Some of the mechanisms controlling hematopoiesis involve cell contacts within the hematopoietic microenvironment formed by the stroma; however, much of the control of blood cell formation is mediated by a group of specific regulatory glycoproteins [1, 2]. These glycoproteins, also known as hematopoietic growth factors or colony-stimulating factors (CSFs), are produced by a variety of cells, and interact with target cells in each of the hematopoietic lineages to stimulate proliferation and differentiation.

Evidence for the existence of a growth factor that stimulates multiple hematopoietic and other lineages was provided by a study of mutations in the mouse genome, at loci known as the *SI,* or steel locus, and at the *W,* or white-spotting locus. Various *W* and *SI* mutations result in defects in the hematopoietic, gonadal, and melanocytic cell lineages. These include a macrocytic anemia resistant to the action of erythropoietin [3], abnormalities in megakaryopoiesis [4], reduced granulopoiesis [5], deficiency in tissue mast cells [6], and impaired development of hematopoietic stem cells. Further experiments have shown that the defect in *W* mutations is intrinsic to the hematopoietic stem cell, while the defect in *SI* mutations is in the marrow stromal-cell environment.

There appears to be no exact equivalent to the *W* and *SI* mutations in humans, but the piebald trait is the likeliest candidate for a disease in humans that is similar to the defect seen in *W* and *SI* mice. Humans expressing the piebald trait have white forelocks of hair and areas of hypomelanosis [7].

George Morstyn
Amgen Inc.
1840 DeHavilland Drive
Thousand Oaks, CA 91320-1789 (USA)


0030–2414/94/0512–0205
$5.00/0

**Table 1.** Stem cell factor: description and actions

| |
|---|
| Native hematopoietic glycoprotein, ligand of c-*kit* receptor, a tyrosine kinase |
| Recombinant human stem cell factor<br>produced in *E. coli* expression system<br>165 amino acids plus N-terminal methionine<br>nonglycosylated<br>exists as a noncovalent dimer<br>molecular weight 36 kD |
| Both native and recombinant forms act in synergy with colony-stimulating factors and interleukins to stimulate both primitive and mature progenitor cells of the hematopoietic system |
| Anticipated actions of recombinant human SCF include:<br>expansion of bone marrow cellularity<br>multilineage stimulation<br>increase in peripheral leukocytes, platelets, erythrocytes, and progenitor cells |

Several groups have demonstrated that the gene product of the *W* locus is the proto-oncogene c-*kit* [8, 9] which is a transmembrane tyrosine kinase receptor.

The molecular identification of the ligand for the c-*kit* receptor was shown to be encoded by the *Sl* locus [10, 11]. It is a glycoprotein, called stem cell factor (SCF), and is also known as steel factor, mast cell growth factor (M-CGF), and c-*kit* ligand. It has a broad range of activities, including effects on a cell at or near the level of the multipotential stem cell as well as on hematopoietic cells that are committed to myeloid, erythroid, and lymphoid lineages. SCF has additional effects on subsets of neuroectodermal-derived and epithelial cells.

## Biochemical Characteristics of SCF

The soluble form of SCF is a glycosylated protein with a molecular weight of approximately 45 kD in its dimeric form, including the carbohydrate moieties [12]. The protein sequence is highly conserved across species with about 83% amino acid homology between murine and human forms, although species-specific molecules are needed for accurate measures of functional activity.

SCF is most abundant in bone-marrow stromal cells and it exists naturally in membrane-bound and soluble forms [13]. The human SCF molecule is encoded by a gene on chromosome 12. There is a 25-amino-acid leader sequence, an extracellular domain of 185 amino acids, a trans-membrane segment of 27 amino acids, and a 36-amino-acid cytoplasmic domain. The soluble form exhibits all three domains. The cDNAs have been identified that encode for the two forms, $SCF^{248}$ and $SCF^{220}$. The extracellular domain of human $SCF^{248}$ cleaves into a 165-amino-acid soluble molecule; $SCF^{220}$ is present only in the membrane-bound form since it lacks exon 6 which is believed to encode for a proteolytic cleavage site necessary for expression of the soluble form [13].

The SCF receptor, c-*kit,* is a class III tyrosine kinase protein receptor. Binding of SCF ligand to the c-*kit* receptor activates its tyrosine kinase activity, resulting in autophosphorylation of tyrosine residues and conformational changes [14]. The human proto-oncogene encoding c-*kit* is on chromosome 4. SCF receptors can be detected in cells that originated in the embryonic neural crest, such as hematopoietic cells, melanocytes, and primordial germ cells. In humans, the SCF receptor is also expressed on some malignant cells, including blast cells in patients with acute myeloid leukemia as well as occasional epithelial malignancies.

SCF was purified in 1989 and the human gene was first cloned at Amgen Inc. (Thousand Oaks, Calif., USA) [10, 12]. Recombinant methionyl human SCF (r-metHuSCF), a noncovalent dimeric protein produced in *Escherichia coli,* bears an additional amino acid (N-terminal methionine) compared with the native form, and is nonglycosylated.

Table 1 describes and summarizes the actions of both native and r-metHuSCF.

## In vitro Biology

SCF appears to act on both lineage-committed and noncommitted progenitor cells in the presence of other CSFs or interleukins (ILs). The role of SCF alone in vitro is very limited, with a modest stimulation of neutrophil colonies. In combination with other factors, SCF has little effect on lineage commitment, with the nature of mature cells generated dependent on the secondary factors.

### *Stem Cells*

Experiments by Bernstein et al. [15] have shown that r-metHuSCF is able to maintain the viability of highly immature progenitor cells and allows them to proliferate in response to other hematopoietic growth factors. The action of SCF appeared to be direct, because accessory cells were not required.

In one series of experiments, highly immature (CD34+) cells were grown in liquid colony culture in the presence of hematopoietic growth factors [IL-3, IL-6, erythropoietin (EPO), granulocyte-macrophage CSF (GM-CSF), or granulocyte CSF (G-CSF)] with and without r-metHuSCF [15]. Colony formation by isolated CD34+ cells was enhanced by the addition of r-metHuSCF. Furthermore, it was found that the enhanced colony growth was most dramatic within a small subpopulation of highly primitive, lineage-uncommitted stem cells (CD34+, lin–). Addition of r-metHuSCF to these cultures resulted in increased numbers of colony-forming cells (CFCs).

The murine high-proliferative-potential (HPP)-CFC is an early hematopoietic progenitor cell with repopulating ability, and is optimally derived from enriched progenitor populations when stimulated with combinations of hematopoietic growth factors [16]. When recombinant rodent (rr)SCF was added at the initiation of a culture, one group reported that it maintained a subset of HPP-CFC for as long as 96 h, which can then be detected following stimulation with other multiple growth factor combinations. It was noted that CSF-1 could only support a much smaller subset of HPP-CFC [17], demonstrating that in a temporal, hierarchical sequence such as the ability of growth factors to sustain HPP-CFC, SCF seems to be an early-acting factor.

Koller et al. [18] found that in perfusion cultures of cord blood mononuclear cells on a preformed irradiated marrow stroma, addition of r-metHuSCF to the combination of IL-3 and IL-6 yielded increases in the number of CFU-GM (18-fold), CFU-Mix (5-fold), and long-term-culture-initiating cells (LTC-IC) (3-fold) compared with cultures that were static and not perfused.

*Progenitor Cells*

In addition to its action on very primitive cells, SCF also has marked effects on committed progenitors. McNiece et al. [16] reported that r-metHuSCF would synergize with GM-CSF, G-CSF, IL-3, and EPO to stimulate progenitors. Although r-metHuSCF alone on human bone marrow cells resulted in no significant colony formation, in the presence of other growth factors, a synergistic increase in colony numbers was seen. These colonies were of increased size compared with expected colony growth without r-metHuSCF, and the morphology of the cells in the colony was predictable from the second growth factor with which r-metHuSCF was combined, demonstrating that r-metHuSCF could directly stimulate progenitor cells of both myeloid and erythroid lineages.

Similar results were reported from Heyworth et al. [19] who found that in soft-agar assays, using both serum-containing and serum-deprived cultures, rrSCF alone promoted the formation of small colonies that contained primarily granulocytic cells with some blast cells also present. Colonies cultured with both IL-3 and rrSCF contained granulocytes, macrophages, and blasts. In serum-deprived cultures, no colonies were formed in the presence of macrophage (M)-CSF, but when M-CSF and r-metHuSCF were combined, large colonies were produced containing predominantly macrophages. Synergistic actions were also noted between recombinant methionyl human G-CSF (r-metHuG-CSF) and rrSCF. When rrSCF was added to colony-forming assays, the amounts of G-CSF and IL-3 required for optimal colony growth were markedly reduced. The results of this study suggest that rrSCF acts directly on highly enriched committed progenitor cells in serum-deprived conditions to promote the survival, proliferation, and development of GM-CFCs.

*B Cells*

It has been proposed that rrSCF promotes the differentiation of pro-B (B220–) to pre-B (B220+) lymphocytic cells; r-metHuSCF has no action on mature B cell function as responsiveness to SCF is lost late in the pre-B stage. McNiece et al. [20] found that r-metHuSCF and IL-7 in combination increased colony numbers of pre-B cell clones in murine bone marrow cell cultures. There was an increased cell proliferation per colony with the combination when compared with either factor alone. SCF alone and in combination with IL-7 stimulated generation of B220+ cells in liquid culture of B220– cells, whereas IL-7 alone had no stimulatory effect on B220– B cells. The authors suggest that r-metHuSCF synergizes with IL-7 to stimulate the proliferation and differentiation of pro-B cells to pre-B cells, which then become responsive to Il-7 alone.

*Mast Cells*

It has been found that SCF is important for the survival, proliferation, and differentiation of mast cells and that it influences all stages of their development. When immature mast cells are cultured with r-metHuSCF, they expand, differentiate, and increase their histamine content.

The in vitro effects of r-metHuSCF on human mast cells from the skin and on peripheral blood basophils was determined by Columbo et al. [21]. r-metHuSCF causes the proliferation of purified human mast cells in culture and may enhance the release of histamine from skin mast cells and peripheral blood basophils at concentrations at or above the normal circulating amount found in human plasma. When CD34+ cells are cultured in the presence of both recombinant human IL-3 (rHuIL-3) and r-metHuSCF, they give rise to cultures containing increased numbers of basophils and mast cells, with the mast cells showing ultrastructural evidence of maturation, although the percentages of basophils and mast cells arising in these cultures remain unchanged [22].

### *Distribution of SCF Receptors on Normal and Malignant Cells*

Pietsch et al. [23] defined a subset of myeloid leukemia cell lines and fresh leukemic blasts that have receptors for SCF and proliferate in response to SCF. This ability to proliferate following stimulation with r-metHuSCF did not appear to correlate with any distinct morphologic type of myeloid leukemic cells as the responding cell lines had different Fab types. The leukemic cell lines that responded to r-metHuSCF expressed 2,300 to 29,000 binding sites per cell. This study suggests that SCF may be an important factor for the growth of myeloid leukemic cells and, if this is so, r-metHuSCF may be able to bring quiescent leukemic cells into cycle, thereby increasing their susceptibility to chemotherapeutic agents.

Broudy et al. [24] studied the response of neoplastic human cells to r-metHuSCF by culturing bone marrow mononuclear cells from 20 patients with newly diagnosed acute myelogenous leukemia as well as cells from two normal volunteers. r-metHuSCF, IL-3, and IL-3 plus r-metHuSCF were used; r-metHuSCF appeared to stimulate colony growth in 7 of the 20 samples, although a statistically significant change in colony numbers was found in only 4 of the 20. Blast cells from all 20 patients had receptors for SCF, and ranged from 600 to 29,000 per cell. A majority of patients also had low-affinity binding sites. This suggests that the SCF receptors on leukemic blast cells may be functional and that SCF might stimulate a proliferative response in these cells; however, there seemed to be no relationship between receptor number and response.

Premalignant cells from patients with myelodysplastic syndromes (MDS) have been studied by Soligo et al. [25]. The effect of r-metHuSCF was evaluated using bone marrow mononuclear cells from 40 patients with MDS in terms of CFU-GM, CFU-GEMM, and BFU-E. r-metHuSCF with GM-CSF and/or IL-3 yielded an approximate 20% increase in the number and size of CFU-GM, but r-metHuSCF, even in combination with other cytokines, never produced a significant increase in cluster formation. Response to r-metHuSCF was mixed, with cells from 22 of the 40 patients showing no response, 13 reaching subnormal or normal BFU-E numbers, and 5 achieving colony numbers comparable with or even greater than normal control cells cultured with r-metHuSCF. The authors believe that these results suggest that there may be a clinical role for r-metHuSCF in the treatment of MDS because of its potent effect on the erythroid series in some patients.

Receptors have also been reported on nonmyeloid cells; for example, Berdel et al. [26] found that r-metHuSCF stimulated the growth of a human glioblastoma cell line expressing the SCF receptor. Of the eight glioblastoma cell lines investigated, however, only one cell line could be stimulated by SCF. The clinical relevance of these observations is uncertain.

### *Ex vivo Cell Expansion and Gene Therapy*

A major application of SCF appears to be for the expansion of progenitor cells and mature cells ex vivo. Haylock et al. [27] reported a greater than 50-fold expansion of progenitor cells and a greater than 200-fold expansion of mature cells. This technology may have a major application for the production of early and mature cells of various lineages to support myelosuppressive chemotherapy.

Severe combined immunodeficiency syndrome (SCIDS) caused by adenosine deaminase (ADA) deficiency was explored as a candidate for genetic correction using bone marrow stem cells [28]. In a Rhesus monkey model, CD34+ cells were isolated from donor animals and seeded onto a stromal cell line engineered to produce the membrane-bound form of SCF to improve the survival and proliferation of human CD34+ cells. The cells were cultured with PGKm-ADA provirus supernatant prior to infusion into irradiated donor animals. In the longest surviving animal (135 days post transplant), approximately 5% of the peripheral blood contained the provirus. Clinical trials have started in humans using the combination of IL-3, IL-6, and SCF ex vivo to introduce retroviral vectors carrying the ADA gene, for example, into hematopoietic progenitor cells from bone marrow or peripheral blood.

## In vivo Biology

A summary of preclinical study results is given in table 2.

*SCF as a Single Agent*

*Rodent Model*

A single intravenous injection of approximately 100 µg/kg rrSCF caused neutrophilia and lymphocytosis as well as the appearance of immature myeloid cells and a few blast cells in the peripheral blood of rats [29]. Unlike some other cytokines, such as G-CSF and GM-CSF [30–35], rrSCF did not cause a decrease in circulating neutrophil numbers. Neutrophil levels became detectably elevated 2 h after the injection, peaked between 4 and 6 h, and subsided between 12 and 24 h. Lymphocytosis was shown to occur at 0.5 h and to subside by 2 h. When the peripheral blood was examined 6 h after administration of rrSCF, there was a significant increase in the absolute numbers of morphologically recognizable early myeloid and erythroid precursor cells and a concurrent decrease in the absolute numbers of mature marrow neutrophils. This suggests that a release of bone marrow neutrophils contributes to the peripheral blood neutrophilia. Mast cells were reported in the peripheral circulation and there appeared to be a systemic increase in embryonic connective-tissue-type, but not mucosal-type, mast cells.

Following daily subcutaneous administration of polyethylene glycol (PEG)-modified rrSCF to normal mice for 21 days, a modest (2- to 3-fold) leukocytosis in pretreatment blood tests occurred [36]. The increase in the leukocyte count was predominantly due to neutrophils, although increases in lymphoid cells were also seen. Reticulocytosis was observed with no changes in hematocrit. During chronic dosing, SCF had no effect on the platelet count; however, an increase in platelets was noted after dosing had ceased [36]. Peripheral blood CFU-S levels increased dramatically during SCF therapy. Bone-marrow cellularity was not consistently altered, but an increase in splenic cellularity occurred due to increased hematopoiesis. A 50-fold increase in IL-3-responsive progenitor cells and a 4- to 6-fold increase in CFU-S was observed in the spleen. These and other observations [37] suggest that an amplification of early hematopoietic cells may occur in vivo in response to SCF [36].

Chow and Hamburger [38] evaluated the ability of SCF to alleviate thrombocytopenia in a murine model of AIDS (MAIDS). The authors concluded that SCF can elevate platelet counts in both thrombocytopenic MAIDS and normal mice and can greatly affect CFU-MK proliferation.

**Table 2.** Preclinical results of studies with SCF

| |
|---|
| In a murine model, SCF pretreatment protected against lethal irradiation. |
| In a canine model, SCF enhanced survival and accelerated hematologic recovery from total body irradiation. |
| In a normal baboon model, 200 µg/kg/day for ≤ 28 days elicited a multilineage response in peripheral counts and increases in bone marrow cellularity. |
| In a normal baboon model, 25–200 µg/kg/day for ≤ 28 days increased circulating progenitor cells up to 300-fold in a dose-dependent manner. |

The radioprotective effects of PEG-modified rrSCF have been studied in mice receiving a lethal dose of total-body irradiation (TBI) [14]. No control mice survived more than 11 days after TBI. In contrast, 30-day survival was 100% in mice (n = 300) receiving rrSCF at 20 and 2 h prior to and 4 h after TBI at 1,150 cGy. Peripheral-blood hematology in SCF-treated mice showed no significant difference compared with the control mice over the first 8 days postirradiation; however, by day 10, significant differences between the rrSCF and control mice were seen in all three cell lines with recovery to normal red blood cell, white blood cell, and platelet values by day 21 occurring in the rrSCF-treated mice. There was also early evidence of marrow hematopoietic recovery (days 5–6) in the rrSCF-treated animals.

*Canine Model*

The effects of recombinant canine (rc)SCF on the hematopoiesis of normal and lethally irradiated dogs was studied by Schuening et al. [39]. Four dogs with intact bone marrow received 200 µg/kg/day for 28 days (intravenously) or 20 days (subcutaneously in two divided doses). All dogs showed at least a 2-fold increase in peripheral blood neutrophil counts beginning about 7 days after initiation of treatment, but there were no effects on hematocrits nor on monocyte, lymphocyte, eosinophil, reticulocyte, or platelet counts.

Ten additional dogs were given 400 cGy TBI without bone marrow infusion. rcSCF was given 200 µg/kg/day subcutaneously in two divided doses for 21 days beginning within 2 h of irradiation. The results from these dogs were compared with those obtained in a previous study of

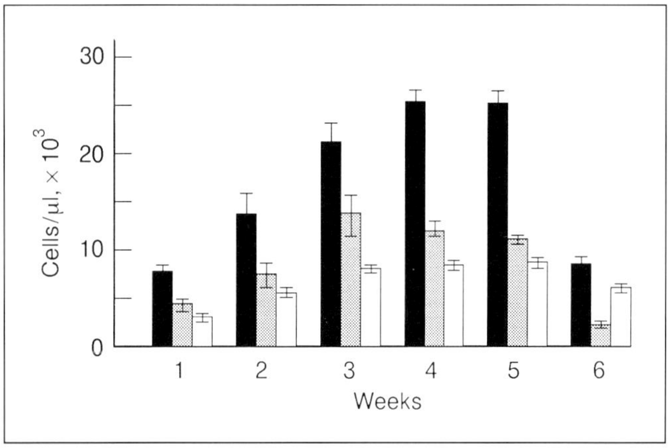


**Fig. 1.** Changes in peripheral blood counts for white blood cells (■), neutrophils (▨) and lymphocytes (□) (means ± SE) for two animals given unmodified SCF and two animals given PEG-SCF (200 μg/kg/day for 28 days as a continuous intravenous infusion). Adapted from Andrews et al. [40].

TBI-induced myelosuppression in five dogs receiving r-metHuG-CSF and seven dogs receiving no hematopoietic growth factor support [39]. Five of the 10 evaluable dogs treated with r-metHuSCF showed complete and sustained hematopoietic recovery and survived. In a previous study, none of the dogs treated without growth factor support survived, whereas four of the five dogs treated with r-metHuG-CSF did.

The duration of neutropenia in the five surviving dogs receiving rcSCF was similar to that in five dogs treated with r-metHuG-CSF. The absolute neutrophil count (ANC) nadir of the r-metHuG-CSF-treated dogs was 15–20 days. Treatment with rcSCF resulted in a significant reduction in the median duration of thrombocytopenia. The median time to recovery of platelets to 50.0 × $10^9$/l was reported to be 33 days post-TBI for the rcSCF-treated dogs and 46 days for the r-metHuG-CSF-treated dogs.

When the radiation dose was increased, treatment with rcSCF allowed hematopoietic recovery in two of seven dogs given 500 cGy TBI, but in none of the five dogs given 600 cGy TBI.

*Primate Model*

The effects of r-metHuSCF on hematopoiesis were determined in two studies of baboons given r-metHuSCF at a dose of 200 μg/kg/day by continuous intravenous infusion for up to 28 days [40, 41]. Animals were observed daily for any abnormal behavior or signs of toxicity. Peripheral blood and bone marrow cells were obtained at intervals during the study to assess the hematopoietic response.

After 3 weeks of dosing, the peripheral white blood cell count increased by 3.9-fold (range 2.9- to 5.3-fold). Neutrophils, lymphocytes, macrophages, eosinophils, and basophils all increased. Reticulocyte counts increased during the early part of dosing, and the red blood cell count and hematocrit increased from the second week of dosing to 2 weeks after dosing. The platelet count remained within the normal range. Bone marrow cellularity increased to between 160 and 200% of baseline after 4 weeks of dosing. A transient decrease was seen in the myeloid:erythroid (M:E) ratio from baseline (5.2:1) to day 7 (1.3:1), with a predominance of immature myeloid and erythroid cells and an increase in megakaryocytes being seen. The M:E ratio and marrow differential returned to normal by the end of dosing on day 28, even though there was a marked increase in cellularity (200% of normal) throughout the period of r-metHuSCF administration. This suggests that r-metHuSCF causes a multilineage increase in marrow cellularity that is different from the changes seen with r-metHuG-CSF or rHuGM-CSF. CFCs and CD34+ cells doubled in the bone marrow and increased up to 300-fold in the peripheral blood [40]. No adverse events or signs of toxicity were noted.

In a second study, three groups of six normal baboons received r-metHuSCF at dosages of 0, 30, or 100 μg/kg/day by subcutaneous injection for 29 days. Peripheral blood hematology and clinical chemistry studies were done [42]. An increase in white blood cells, predominantly neutrophils and lymphocytes, occurred in a dose-dependent fashion after 10 days of treatment (fig. 1). The hematocrit was increased at several timepoints during dosing in both the 30 and 100 μg/kg/day groups. Platelet counts did not significantly increase in the r-metHuSCF-treated groups. No adverse events were noted during the study.

In further work, Andrews et al. [41] examined the ability of r-metHuSCF to stimulate the circulation of cells that can engraft and rescue lethally irradiated baboons. In this latter study, peripheral blood mononuclear cells from untreated control animals and from animals treated for 10 days with 200 μg/kg/day r-metHuSCF were isolated by leukapheresis and the cells were cryopreserved. Following a single dose of 10.2 Gy TBI, 1 × $10^8$–1.04 × $10^8$/kg cryopreserved mononuclear cells were transplanted into all animals. All three animals receiving r-metHuSCF-mobilized cells responded with trilineage engraftment verified by bone marrow biopsy. The mean times to a white blood cell count >0.5 × $10^9$/l, white blood cell count >1.0 ×

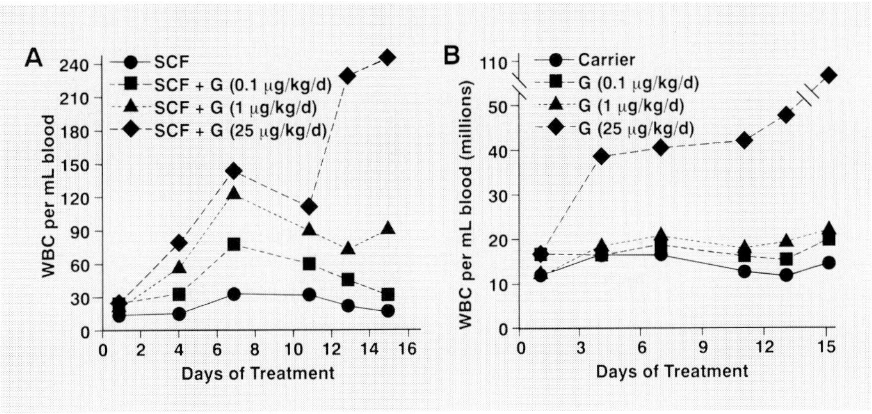


**Fig. 2. A.** The changes in peripheral blood nucleated cell count during treatment with PEG-rrSCF (100 μg/kg/day) either alone or in combination with r-metHuG-CSF (G) at 0.1, 1, and 25 μg/kg/day. **B** The effects of r-metHuG-CSF alone on blood leukocytes. Adapted from Molineux et al. [36].

$10^9$/l, and to an ANC >0.5 × $10^9$/l were 15, 19, and 19 days, respectively. Two of the three animals survived with normal blood counts for more than 115 and 180 days, while the third died of infection on day 32. Three other animals were transplanted with cells pheresed without mobilization by r-metHuSCF. At necropsy 13, 28, and 38 days following transplant, it was noted that all three had continued aplasia.

A potential basis for adverse events was revealed by Galli et al. [43] in subcutaneous administration for 21 days to cynomolgus monkeys. The results showed that SCF increased the number of mast cells in many areas of the body. There were no adverse consequences reported for the monkeys, and when treatment was stopped, the mast cell numbers returned quickly to nearly pretreatment values.

*SCF in Combination with Other Cytokines*

In vivo studies have confirmed in vitro observations that SCF potentiates the effects of other hematopoietic growth factors [29, 36, 44]. It has been shown that the combination of rrSCF and r-metHuG-CSF induces a greater-than-additive increase in blood neutrophils and circulating CFU-S when given to normal mice [36]. This synergy was dependent on the dose of G-CSF (fig. 2).

In another study, rrSCF and r-metHuG-CSF injected for 1 week in rats caused a synergistic increase in mature bone marrow neutrophils, accompanied by an approximately 4-fold decrease in erythroid and a greater than 10-fold decrease in lymphoid marrow elements [29]. The spleens of the same rats showed increased granulopoiesis as well as increased erythropoiesis as compared with the spleens of rats treated with either of the growth factors alone. The combination of rrSCF and r-metHuG-CSF caused a greater than additive increase in the rate of release of bone marrow neutrophils into the circulation, and caused a synergistic peripheral neutrophilia of 4- to 17-fold compared to the use of either agent alone. This became most apparent after 4 days of treatment.

In vivo daily administration of rrSCF and rHuGM-CSF also produced a synergistic increase in bone marrow neutrophils, but not the striking synergistic increase in circulating neutrophils observed with rrSCF plus r-metHuG-CSF [29]. Colony-forming assays of all experimental groups showed a synergistic increase in CFU-GM in the bone marrow, but not in peripheral blood, after coincubation with PEG-rrSCF plus rHuGM-CSF. This effect was not seen when rHuGM-CSF was used alone.

Studies by Briddell et al. [44] examined the ability of PEG-rrSCF, r-metHuG-CSF, and a combination of the two factors to mobilize peripheral blood progenitor cells (PBPC) with marrow-repopulating ability in mice. Splenectomized mice were injected intravenously with rrSCF at 200 μg/kg/day for 7 days and the peripheral blood harvested by cardiac puncture. A 5-fold increase in peripheral white blood cell numbers resulted, compared with control mice. Although a cell dose of 10 × $10^6$ low-density mononuclear cells (LDMNC) from normal BDFI mice was required to save lethally irradiated mice, as low as 0.25 × $10^6$ LDMNC from rrSCF-treated mice resulted in 100% survival. Marked increases in circulating mature (CFU-GM) and primitive (HPP-CFC) progenitors were obtained in rrSCF-treated compared with control mice [44].

As r-metHuG-CSF has previously been shown to mobilize PBPC, the effect of combined rrSCF and r-metHuG-CSF treatment of splenectomized mice was examined. A greater-than-additive increase in circulating

**Table 3.** Comparison of PBPC mobilization by rrSCF, r-metHuG-CSF, and a combination of the two factors

| Drug | Dose µg/kg | Peripheral white blood cells × $10^6$/l | CFU-GM per milliliter | HPP-CFC per milliliter | Survival % |
|---|---|---|---|---|---|
| rrSCF | 25 | 24.65±2.21 | 13,311 | 3,081 | 40 |
| r-metHuG-CSF | 200 | 49.26±4.78 | 36,108 | 10,492 | 30 |
| rrSCF | 25 | 76.90±7.49 | 178,408 | 22,532 | 80 |
| + r-metHuG-CSF | 200 | | | | |

Number in each group = 10.

LDMNC, GM-CFC, and HPP-CFC was obtained compared with mice treated with rrSCF or r-metHuG-CSF alone. In three separate experiments, the mobilization potentials of optimal doses of r-metHuG-CSF (200 µg/kg/day for 7 days), low doses of rrSCF (25 µg/kg for 7 days), and combined administration of the two factors have been compared. Data from a typical experiment are summarized in table 3. These data demonstrate that mice treated with the combination of rrSCF (25 µg/kg/day) and r-metHuG-CSF (200 µg/kg/day) had approximately 1.5-fold higher numbers of circulating white blood cells, 5-fold higher CFU-GM, 2-fold higher HPP-CFC, and greater than 5-fold higher numbers of cells with in vivo repopulating ability compared with mice treated with r-metHuG-CSF alone (200 µg/kg/day) [44].

## *Clinical Studies*

Clinical experience with r-metHuSCF is presently in the very early stages.

### *Non-Small Cell Lung Cancer Study*

A phase I trial of r-metHuSCF in previously untreated patients with advanced non-small cell lung cancer is in progress to determine safety and hematological efficacy when given before and after myelosuppressive chemotherapy [45]. r-metHuSCF was given subcutaneously for 14 days at doses of 10, 25, or 50 µg/kg/day followed by a 14-day observation period, then chemotherapy with etoposide and carboplatin and another 14 daily doses of r-metHuSCF. The administration of r-metHuSCF was associated with a more rapid rebound of white blood cell and platelet counts postchemotherapy compared with those of control patients.

In this same study, peripheral blood samples were collected serially in the prechemotherapy stage, and bone marrow samples were collected on days 1 and 14 for progenitor cell analysis [46]. There was evidence of a dose-dependent increase in the number of circulating CFU-GM and BFU-E. Peak hematopoietic progenitor cell mobilization was observed between days 11 and 14. The results support the preclinical data that r-metHuSCF may be a promising agent for progenitor cell mobilization.

### *Breast Cancer Study*

Preliminary data from an on-going phase I study have been reported by Demetri et al. [47] in 21 patients with stage IIIB or IV breast cancer receiving r-metHuSCF alone in the prechemotherapy stage, and in cycles 2–6 of chemotherapy with cyclophosphamide and doxorubicin. Patients were randomized to receive either r-metHuSCF at dosages of 10, 25, and 50 µg/kg/day or no r-metHuSCF as a parallel comparative group. The ANCs showed an upward trend in the prechemotherapy stage with no marked changes in platelets or red blood cell variables. Administration of r-metHuSCF was found to mobilize leukopoietic progenitor cells into the peripheral blood.

Punch biopsies of skin were taken over the posterior iliac crest before and after r-metHuSCF administration to quantify the number of mast cells [48]. It was reported that r-metHuSCF for 14 days resulted in a doubling of dermal mast cells as well as a slight increase in the amount of histamine metabolite excreted into the urine.

Bone marrow biopsies of seven of these breast cancer patients were evaluated before and after 14 days of treatment with r-metHuSCF at doses of 10–50 µg/kg/day [49]. After treatment, bone marrow cellularity increased up to 1.6-fold with an increased proportion of progenitor cells and unchanged relative frequencies of other marrow cells. There was also an increase in the CD34+ bone marrow progenitor cells from 0.9 to 1.8%. Bone marrow fibrosis and macrophage increases were not noted, but the white blood cell count increased 1.3- to 3.6-fold in all seven

**Table 4.** Clinical potential of r-metHuSCF

| |
|---|
| Support of standard-dose chemotherapy |
| Use in bone marrow transplantation |
| marrow expansion before harvest |
| marrow expansion before and after transplantation to accelerate engraftment |
| Mobilization of PBPC |
| Treatment of aplastic anemia and other bone marrow failure syndromes |
| Adjunctive therapy in HIV infection |

patients. Other cell types showing increases included neutrophils, reticulocytes, and platelets.

*Side Effects*

The most frequently observed adverse events in the phase I trials were dermatologic reactions localized to injection sites. Symptoms included erythema, pruritus, and swelling. While doses of 10 μg/kg/day appeared to be well tolerated, doses of 50 μg/kg/day produced generalized rash, urticaria, in some cases cough and in other cases upper-respiratory symptoms such as throat tightening, possibly due to mast cell degranulation.

*Pharmacokinetics*

The pharmacokinetics of r-metHuSCF were investigated in 24 lung or breast cancer patients who received daily subcutaneous doses of 10, 25, or 50 μg/kg for 14 days [50]. Blood samples were obtained at 12 timepoints up to 24 h following doses 1 and 14. The mean area under the curve (AUC) on day 1 increased in proportion to the dose (78, 219, and 368 ng · h/ml, respectively), and at each dose level, the AUC increased about 2-fold from day 1 to day 14. The $C_{max}$ showed a similar dose relationship as the AUC. $T_{max}$ occurred between 13 and 15 h on day 1 and between 4 and 10 h on day 14. Trough concentrations pre- and 24 h post-dose on day 14 were nearly equal suggesting that the steady-state concentration had been reached by day 14.

*Summary of Clinical Experience*

rmetHuSCF has shown promising biologic activity in expanding the progenitor pool in the bone marrow and peripheral blood. It appears to be tolerated without generalized side effects at doses of 10 μg/kg. Higher doses (50 μg/kg/day) have resulted in systemic allergic-like reactions in some patients.

Table 4 summarizes the clinical potential of r-metHuSCF.

## Conclusions

SCF acts at multiple stages of hematopoiesis. It has in vitro multilineage effects and acts in synergy with other factors. Early clinical results suggest that doses of 10 μg/kg/day or less given subcutaneously are well tolerated. At high doses, adverse events, possibly related to the effects of r-metHuSCF on mast cells, are seen.

r-metHuSCF has major clinical potential because of its synergy with other growth factors. Potentially useful combinations of r-metHuSCF may include those with r-metHuG-CSF, EPO, IL-6, and IL-7, the synergy between γ-metHuSCF and γ-metHUG-CSF in the mobilization of PBPC demonstrated in the rodent model suggest that low doses of r-metHuSCF may greatly enhance the progenitor-cell-mobilizing properties of r-metHuG-CSF.

## References


1 Stanley ER, Jubinsky PT: Factors affecting the growth and differentiation of haemopoietic cells in culture. Clin Haematol 1984;13:329–348.
2 Metcalf D: The granulocyte-macrophage colony-stimulating factor. Science 1985;229:16–22.
3 Bernstein SE, Russell ES, Keighley G: Two hereditary mouse anemias (Sl/Sl$^d$ and W/W$^v$) deficient in response to erythropoietin. Ann NY Acad Sci 1968;149:475–485.
4 Ebbe S, Phalen E, Stohlman F: Abnormalities of megakaryocytes in S1-S1d mice. Blood 1973; 42:865–871.
5 Ruscetti F, Boggs DK, Torok BJ, Boggs SS: Reduced blood and marrow neutrophils and granulocyte colony forming cells in Sl/Sl$^d$ mice. Soc Exp Biol Med 1976;1528:398–402.
6 Kitamura Y, Go S, Hatanaka K: Decrease of mast cells in W/Wv mice and their increase by bone marrow transplantation. Blood 1978;52: 447–452.
7 Hulten MA, Honeyman MM, Mayne AJ, Tarlow MJ: Homozygosity in piebald trait. J Med Genet 1987;24:568–571.
8 Chabot B, Stephenson DA, Chapman VM, Besmer P, Bernstein A: The protooncogene c-*kit* encoding a transmembrane tyrosine kinase receptor maps to the mouse W locus. Nature 1988;335:88–89.
9 Geissler EN, Rayan MA, Houseman KE: The dominant spotting (W) locus of the mouse encodes for the c-*kit* proto-oncogene. Cell 1988; 55:185–192.

10 Zsebo KM, Williams DA, Geissler EN, et al: Stem cell factor is encoded at the sI locus of the mouse and is the ligand for the c-*kit* tyrosine kinase receptor. Cell 1990;63:213–224.
11 Martin FH, Suggs SV, Langley KE, et al: Primary structure and functional expression of rat and human stem cell factor cDNAs. Cell 1990; 63:203–211.
12 Zsebo KM, Wypch J, McNiece IK, et al: Identification, purification, and biological characterization of hematopoietic stem cell factor from buffalo rat liver-conditioned medium. Cell 1990;63:195–201.
13 Toksoz D, Zsebo KM, Smith KA, et al: Support of human hematopoiesis in long-term bone marrow cultures by murine stromal cells selectively expressing the membrane-bound and secreted forms of the human homolog of the steel gene product, stem cell factor. Proc Natl Acad Sci USA 1992;89:7350–7354.
14 Zsebo KM, Smith KA, Hartley CA, et al: Radioprotection of mice by recombinant rat stem cell factor; Proc Natl Acad Sci USA 1992;89: 9464–9468.
15 Bernstein ID, Andrews RG, Zsebo KM: Recombinant human stem cell factor enhances the formation of colonies by CD34+ and CD34+lin− cells, and the generation of colony-forming cell progeny from CD34+lin− cells cultured with interleukin-3, granulocyte colony-stimulating factor, or granulocyte-macrophage colony-stimulating factor. Blood 1991;77: 2316–2321.
16 McNiece IK, Langley KE, Zsebo KM: Recombinant human stem cell factor synergises with GM-CSF, G-CSF, IL-3 and Epo to stimulate human progenitor cells of the myeloid and erythroid lineages. Exp Hematol 1991;19:226–232.
17 Lowry PA, Whitefield P, Deacon D, Quesenberry PJ: Grwoth factors direct proliferation of murine HPP-CFC in a temporal hierarchy. Blood 1992;80:676a.
18 Koller MR, Bender JG, Miller WM, Papoutsakis ET: Expansion of primitive human hematopoietic progenitors in a profusion bioreactor system with IL-3, IL-6 and stem cell factor. Biotechnology, in press.
19 Heyworth CM, Whetton AD, Nicholls S, Zsebo K, Dexter TM: Stem cell factor directly stimulates the development of enriched granulocyte-macrophage colony-forming cells and promotes the effects of other colony-stimulating factors. Blood 1992;80:2230–2236.
20 McNiece IK, Langley KE, Zsebo KM: The role of recombinant stem cell factor in early B cell development. J Immunol 1991;146:3785–3790.
21 Columbo M, Horowitz EM, Botana LM, et al: The human recombinant c-*kit* receptor ligand, rhSCF, induces mediator release from human cutaneous mast cells and enhances IgE-dependent mediator release from both skin mast cells and peripheral blood basophils. J Immunol 1992;149:599–608.
22 Kirschenbaum AS, Goff JP, Kessler SW, et al: Effect of IL-3 and stem cell factor on the appearance of human basophils and mast cells from CD34+ pluripotent progenitor cells. J Immunol 1992;149:599–608.
23 Pietsch T, Kyas U, Stefens U, et al: Effects of human stem cell factor (c-*kit* ligand) on proliferation of myeloid leukemia cells: Heterogeneity in response and synergy with other hematopoietic growth factors. Blood 1992;80:1199–1206.
24 Broudy VC, Smith FO, Lin N, Zsebo K, Egrie J, Bernstein ID: Blasts from patients with acute myelogenous leukemia express functional receptors for stem cell factor. Blood 1992;80:60–67.
25 Soligo D, Servida F, Morgutti M, et al: Effect of recombinant stem cell factor on colony formation and long term bone marrow cultures (LTBMC) in 40 patients with myelodysplastic syndrome. Blood 1992;80:100a.
26 Berdel WE, de Vos S, Maurer J, et al: Recombinant human stem cell factor stimulates the growth of a human glioblastoma cell line expressing c-*kit* protooncogene. Cancer Res 1992; 52:3498–3502.
27 Haylock DN, To LB, Dowse TL, Juttner CA, Simmons PJ: Ex vivo expansion and maturation of peripheral blood CD34+ cells into the myeloid lineage. Blood 1992;80:1405–1412.
28 Bodine D, Moritz T, Luskey B, et al: Expression of the adenosine deaminase (ADA) gene after transduction into Rhesus monkey repopulating stem cells. Blood 1992;80:279a.
29 Ulich TR, del Castillo J, Yi ES, et al: Hematologic effects of stem cell factor in vivo and in vitro in rodents. Blood 1991;78:645–650.
30 Sheridan WP, Morstyn G, Wolf M, et al: Granulocyte colony-stimulating fator and neutrophil recovery after high-dose chemotherapy and autologous bone marrow transplantation. Lancet 1989;2:891–895.
31 Morstyn G, Campbell L, Lieschke G, et al: Treatment of chemotherapy-induced neutropenia by subcutaneously administered granulocyte colony-stimulating factor with optimization of dose and duration of therapy. J Clin Oncol 1989;7:1554–1562.
32 Morstyn G, Lieschke GJ, Sherican W, Layton J, Cebon J, Fox RM: Clinical experience with recombinant human granulocyte colony-stimulating factor and granulocyte macrophage colony-stimulating factor; Semin Hematol 1989;26: 9–13.
33 Lieschke GJ, Burgess AW: Granulocyte colony-stimulating factor and granulocyte-macrophage colony-stimulating factor; N Engl J Med 1992;327:28–35.
34 Lieschke GJ, Burgess AW: Granulocyte colony-stimulating factor and granulocyte-macrophage colony-stimulating factor. N Engl J Med 1992;327:99–106.
35 Demetri GD, Spertini O, Pratt ES, et al: GM-CSF and G-CSF have different effects on expression of the neutrophil adhesion receptors LAM-1 & CD11b. Blood 1990;76:178A.
36 Molineux A, Migdalska A, Szmitkowski M, et al: The effects on hematopoiesis of recombinant stem cell factor (ligand for c-*kit*) administered to mice either alone or in combination with granulocyte colony-stimulating factor. Blood 1991;78:961–966.
37 Bodine DM, Seidel NE, Zsebo KM, Orlic D: In vivo administration of stem cell factor to mice increases the absolute number of pluripotent hematopoietic stem cells. Blood 1992;80:39a.
38 Chow FPR, Hamburger AW: Effects of in vivo administration of stem cell factor on thrombopoiesis in normal and immunodeficient mice. Exp Hematol, in press.
39 Schuening FG, Applebaum FR, Deeg HJ, et al: Effects of recombinant canine stem cell factor, a c-*kit* ligand, and recombinant granulocyte colony-stimulating factor on hematopoietic recovery after otherwise lethal total body irradiation. Blood 1993;81:20–26.
40 Andrews RG, Knitter GH, Bartelmez SH, et al: Recombinant human stem cell factor, a c-*kit* ligand, stimulates hematopoiesis in nonhuman primates. Blood 1991;78:1975–1980.
41 Andrews RG, Bensinger WI, Knitter GH, Bernstein ID, Appelbaum FR, Zsebo KM: The ligand for c-*kit* stimulates the circulation of cells that engraft lethally irradiated baboons. Blood 1992;80:2715–2720.
42 Rosen B, Catchatourian R, Egrie J, et al: The in vivo effects of recombinant human stem cell factor (rh-SCF) on hematopoiesis in nonhuman primates. Blood 1990;76:163a.
43 Galli SJ, Iemura A, Garlick DS, Gamba-Vitalo C, Zsebo KM, Andrews RG: Reversible expansion of primate mast cell populations in vivo by stem cell factor. J Clin Invest 1993;91:148–152.
44 Briddell R, Hartley C, Moss S, McNiece I: The role of stem cell factor in mobilization of peripheral blood progenitor cells (PBPC) with marrow repopulating ability in mice. Blood 1992;80:38a.
45 Crawford J, Lau D, Erwin R, Rich W, McGuire B, Meyers F: A phase I trial of recombinant methionyl human stem cell factor (SCF) in patients (pts) with advanced non-small cell lung carcinoma (NSCLC) (abstract). Proc ASCO 12:135.
46 Kurtzberg J, Meyers F, McGuire B, Crawford J: Mobilization of peripheral blood progenitor cells in patients given recombinant methionyl human stem cell factor (abstract). Proc AACR 34:211.
47 Demetri G, Costa J, Hayes D, et al: A phase I trial of recombinant methionyl human stem cell factor (SCF) in patients with advanced breast carcinoma pre- and post-chemotherapy (chemo) with cyclophosphamide (C) and doxorubicin (A) (abstract). Proc AACR 34:217.
48 Costa JJ, Demetri GD, Hayes DF, Merica EA, Menchaca DM, Galli SJ: Increased skin mast cells and urine methyl histamine in patients receiving recombinant methionyl human stem cell factor (abstract). Proc AACR 34:211.
49 Orazi A, Gordon MS, Neiman RS, et al: Bone marrow effects of recombinant methionyl human stem cell factor (SCF) in patients with normal hematopoiesis (abstract). Proc AACR 34: 465.
50 Young J, Crawford J, Gordon M, et al: Pharmacokinetics (pk) of recombinant methionyl human stem cell factor (SCF) in patients (pts) with lung or breast cancer in phase I trials (abstract). Proc AACR 34:217.

**Supplement Issue**
Included in subscription

**European Urology** (ISSN 0302–2838), **Vol. 20, Suppl. 2 (1991)**
Editor: C.C. Schulman, Brussels

# Changing Attitutes in the Treatment of Benign Prostatic Hyperplasia: The Role of 5α-Reductase Inhibition

**Editors:**
**Fritz H. Schröder, Rotterdam;**
**Adolphe Steg, Paris**

Proceedings of Two Symposia in Nice, November 11, 1989 and Amsterdam, June 14, 1990

International experts on benign prostatic hyperplasia (BPH) present the-state-of-the-art of what is currently known of the epidemiology, pathophysiology, diagnosis and treatment of BPH. Epidemiologic data are examined, such as the relationship of BPH to prostate cancer. Focus is also on the importance of objective assessment of both irritative and obstructive symptoms of BPH and on the evaluation of the advantages and disadvantages of various imaging techniques. Though surgery is currently considered the optimal treatment, a variety of new therapeutic approaches are investigated with special attention paid to the new therapeutic class of 5α-reductase inhibitors. Also discussed are quality of life issues to be considered when assessing the patient with BPH. This publication will increase the scope of practical knowledge relevant to BPH and help readers to gain further insight into promising new dimensions of treatment options.

**Fields of Interest**

Urology, Oncology, Pharmacology

**Contents**



**Changing Attitutes in the Treatment of Benign Prostatic Hyperplasia: The Role of 5α-Reductase Inhibition**
Proceedings of Two Symposia in Nice, November 11, 1989 and Amsterdam, June 14, 1990
'European Urology', Vol. 20, Suppl. 2 (1991)
Editors: Schröder, F.H. (Rotterdam); Steg, A. (Paris)
IV + 92 p., 40 fig., 28 tab., soft cover, 1991
SFr. 34.– / DM 41.– / US$ 27.25
Prices subject to change. DM price for FRG, US$ price for USA only
ISBN 3-8055-5516-4

KI 92039

KARGER